Laugh and Learn About Childbirth

SHERI BAYLES, RN, BSN

www.laughandlearn.com

For information: www.laughandlearn.com
                 info@laughandlearn.com

Cover Design by Mario Geissler
Book Design by www.popshopstudio.com
Illustrations by Claudia Vitt and John Arzayus

ISBN-10: 0-615-27545-1
ISBN-13: 978-0-615-27545-1

10 9 8 7 6 5 4 3 2

Dedication

To Rob, who has been there from the very beginning of this journey. You are the BEST husband, father and friend a woman could ever wish for. I love you forever.

To Aaron and Zachary, my real life began the day you were born. Thank you for giving me my best credential yet: Mother of twin boys. I love you with all my heart.

To Mom and Dad who taught me that humor is a great teaching tool. I know you are always watching from up above. You are the reason I am the woman I am today. I love you and miss you.

Acknowledgements

This book would not have been possible without the tremendous support and efforts of my two business partners, Gene Cernilli and Mario Geissler. Gene, my biggest fan who convinced me from the very beginning that we could do this. And Mario, who put us on the map.

Many thanks to Tami Coyne who helped me tremendously and to Heather Kern who beautifully designed this book.

I also want to thank all the many Lamaze Moms and Dads I have taught over the years who all asked me when I was going to write a book and all those who contributed to my many stories in it. I could not have done this without you.

Contents

Introduction

My motto has always been that no matter how it happens, the delivery should result in both a healthy mother and baby. And the Lamaze method would have been just as helpful to me even if more medical intervention had been necessary.

— Sheri Bayles

If you are a typical **first time expectant mother** or father you are probably a bit scared and nervous about the process of childbirth. This is completely normal! Anytime we humans venture into un-charted waters we feel a bit off balance. **The good news is that unlike some adventures into the unknown, labor and delivery is not an unsolved mystery.** Women have been giving birth since the beginning of mankind - which has given us plenty of time to compile all the information you'll need to successfully give birth to your beautiful baby!

To be fair, some of your anxiety might be the result of the medical establishment that has promoted a fear-based approach to childbirth, which has transformed a natural and beautiful process into a medical procedure. Not all doctors are guilty of this, of course, but the key to overcoming this fear and anxiety is for YOU to take charge of your birthing experience. For years, women have handed their labor and delivery experience over to their physicians and are often unsatisfied with the results. This is your labor and your delivery. You will remember it for the rest of your life. The decisions you make can often impact the outcome. Knowledge is power! The more you know, the better it is for all involved. Relax and trust the wisdom of your body. Empower yourself by asking for what you need, whether that means more information or better support and use the knowledge contained in this book to help yourself prepare for the life-altering event called childbirth.

I'm Sheri Bayles and I'm the author of this book and the instructor on the *Laugh and Learn About Childbirth* DVDs. And, luckily for you, I'm well qualified for the job. I am an RN who has worked at New York Presbyterian Hospital in New York City for 24 years. As an OB/GYN nurse, Lamaze Certified Childbirth Educator, and International Board Certified Lactation Consultant, I've taught over 4,000 couples the Lamaze philosophy. (Yes, even some celebrities, but my lips are sealed).

More importantly, however, I'm a mother. For most people, labor is a private affair involving one's spouse or partner and maybe a doula[1] in addition to the doctor or midwife. For me, it was more like an Off-Broadway production. Countless numbers of colleagues from the hospital stopped by to offer encouragement, but what they really wanted to know was whether I was going to be able to walk my talk and "hee-hee"[2] my way through the pain of labor. I'm proud to say that the Lamaze techniques did indeed work for most of my labor, but I did need pain medication to successfully deliver my twin sons vaginally.

I feel fortunate and happy that my beautiful boys were born as naturally as was possible for me at the time. (I'm equally proud that my husband was a huge support during the blessed event,

---

[1] A labor Doula is a woman experienced in childbirth whose job is to give emotional and physical support to the mother before, during and after labor and delivery. She also functions as an informational resource to the mother and father-to-be regarding the childbirth process.

[2] A Lamaze breathing technique. Don't worry—I'll teach you all about it in the pages that follow!

although, like most partners, he was nervous going in.) Had my boys been delivered by a Cesarean section, it would have been OK as well. My motto has always been that no matter how it happens, the delivery should result in both a healthy mother and baby. And the Lamaze method would have been just as helpful to me even if more medical intervention had been necessary.

What I love about Lamaze, as well as all childbirth education, is that it's not intended to tell a woman what to do. Using the Lamaze philosophy and techniques doesn't mean that you can't have an epidural[3] if you feel you really need it. Rather, it is designed to empower a woman's own natural wisdom about childbirth and provide information, options, coping strategies and support. It can also help spouses and partners become part of the process.

The term "natural childbirth" is now a household word, but way back in the dark ages of the 1950's and early 1960's, most American women gave birth under total anesthesia and breast-feeding was discouraged. All of that has changed thanks to the pioneering work of several forward-thinking people who wisely put the woman back into the child-birthing equation.

In the 1930's, British obstetrician Dr. Grantly Dick-Read wrote a landmark book called *Childbirth without Fear: The Principles and Practice of Natural Childbirth* that was the forerunner of the natural childbirth movement. Then, in the early 1950's, Fernand Lamaze and Pierre Vellay, two French obstetricians, created the Lamaze method after traveling to Russia where they were impressed by Ivan Pavlov's work[4] with conditioned response.

At the time, the core of the Lamaze method involved the use of distraction techniques during contractions, including the famous hee-hee's. No, Lamaze didn't make child birth pain-free, but it did make it manageable — which allowed both a woman and her partner to truly experience, rather than fear, the most beautiful and mystifying of all human experiences.

As the years have progressed, so has the Lamaze organization. Although most people who come to my classes still believe the focus of the

www.laughandlearn.com

---

3   The type of anesthesia used to control pain while remaining fully awake and aware during childbirth.
4   Yes, the same Ivan Pavlov most well known for his work with dogs. While studying the physiological effects of digestion, Pavlov noticed that the dogs could be conditioned to salivate on demand by introducing a stimulus before feeding. The story goes that Pavlov would ring a bell right before feeding time. Eventually, the dogs began to associate the ringing of the bell with food and would salivate at the sound regardless of whether there was any food present.

class is on breathing, they are surprised to find that we have updated our curriculum and made it more user-friendly. We no longer call it "natural childbirth"; instead, we have replaced it with "normal birth". In addition, the term, "Lamaze method" has changed to the "Lamaze philosophy". We believe that women have their own coping mechanisms and must find their own comfort zone. If that includes breathing, great! However, it is not a prerequisite for a normal birth.

As I said at the beginning, I've worked with over 4,000 couples - all of them unique in their own ways and all of them in the same exact boat. Soon, you'll either be delivering your baby into the world or watching and assisting with the birth and you need to be ready to handle it. No matter your personality type or your physical fitness level, labor and delivery are things that every woman can do and every partner can assist with by giving their support through the entire journey into the unknown, including childbirth class! The key to a wonderful labor and delivery is faith in the body's infinite wisdom, combined with knowledge and information about the process itself – and a great sense of humor.

So let's get started.

The key to a wonderful
    labor and delivery is faith in
the body's infinite wisdom,
    combined with knowledge
and information about the
            process itself – and a
great sense of humor.

Chapter One

If you want to be a real smarty-pants, at
36 or 37 weeks you can go into the doctor
or midwife's office and ask, "So what's the
pelvic station of my baby?"

— Sheri Bayles

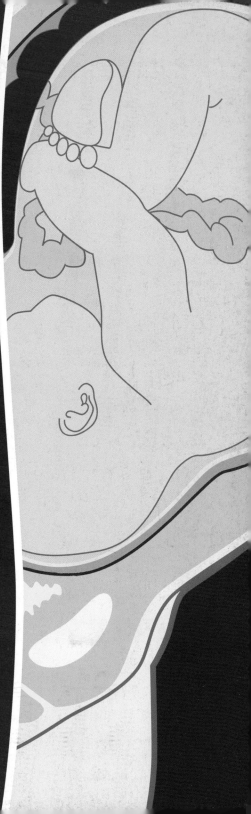

Anatomy And Preliminary Signs of Labor

So you and your partner are starting out on a journey, and you want to consult a map. Ok, I know how you men feel about asking for directions, but since most of you can't tell the difference between a bladder and a fallopian tube, you may want to consult this one. And when it comes to childbirth, the map we need to study is the female body. So, before getting into the preliminary signs of labor, let's take a few moments to get an anatomical feel for what is going on for both mother and baby right before birth.

Pelvic Station

When delivered vaginally, the baby must pass through three areas of the mother's bony pelvis, which forms a cradle of sorts for the baby. The location of the baby's head within the pelvis is called the pelvic station.

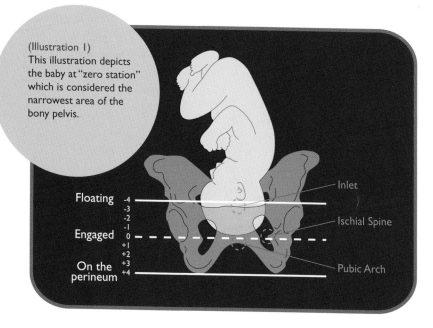

(Illustration 1)
This illustration depicts the baby at "zero station" which is considered the narrowest area of the bony pelvis.

Floating -4
           -3
           -2
           -1
Engaged   0
           +1
           +2
On the   +3
perineum   +4

Inlet

Ischial Spine

Pubic Arch

Not that you have to memorize any of this, but the first area is called the *inlet* and is located at the top of the pubic arch at the -4 station. This is the area where the baby has the most freedom of movement and can create nights of entertainment

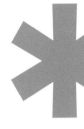

watching the belly move. During labor, the baby passes through the *diagonal conjugate*, which begins at the bottom of the pubic arch and continues straight back to the tailbone (also known as your coccyx) at the very bottom of the spine. The last area and the most important is called the *outlet* (not to be confused with discount clothing and shoes) and is the narrowest area of the pelvis. It is measured by the two boney prominences (points) called ischial spines and is known as "0" (zero) station.

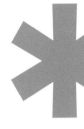

When the baby is floating, moms get kicked in the stomach and in the lungs, and many face the morning with dark circles under their eyes due to a loss of sleep because of the movement.

The stations above the ischial spines are referred to as the *minus stations* and the stations below are called the *plus stations*. Up until 36 weeks (four weeks before your due date), the baby is "floating" at or above the -4 station. When the baby is floating, moms get kicked in the stomach and in the lungs, and many face the morning with dark circles under their eyes due to a loss of sleep because of the movement. Some expectant parents tell me their baby does a lot of what feels like flipping; however, babies don't do summersaults or triple axels in their mother's belly. They move around on an axis, which is why moms get kicked in different areas of the body. Somewhere between 36 - 38 weeks, the baby begins to drop into a -3, -2, or -1 station. This is where the baby will stay until labor begins, at which point the uterine muscle pushes the baby down even further. That dropping is called engagement and there is no ring involved.

In the 1960's, the average baby weighed between six and seven pounds. When I first started teaching in the 1980's, they were seven to eight, but today, the average weight is between eight and nine pounds, primarily because thankfully, women are no longer smoking or drinking through their pregnancies. Smoking is the number one deterrent of fetal growth. Women are also told to gain more weight in their pregnancies than their mothers were advised. Believe it or not, some of your mothers were

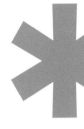

put on Weight Watchers diets during their pregnancies. The overall weight gain is leading to bigger and healthier babies; however, sometimes the mother's pelvic structure cannot accommodate a bigger baby, or in some cases, the woman's position during labor does not allow the baby to move down. Perhaps in the future, with nature on our side, the pelvis will adapt and easily accommodate a larger baby. Now, however, we often hold our breath in the birthing room until the baby moves past the zero station to +1, which means that the largest part of the baby, the head, has just fit through the narrowest area of the pelvis. At the +2 and +3 stations, the baby is in the vagina and at +4 the baby is at the opening of the vagina and ready to be born.

If you want to be a real smarty-pants, at 36 or 37 weeks you can go into the doctor or midwife's office and ask, "So what's the pelvic station of my baby?" The doctor or midwife will then usually ask you "So when did you start reading Sheri Bayles' book?" All joking aside, 36 weeks is an important landmark because in my experience, if the baby doesn't drop into the pelvis within the next two weeks (by 38 weeks), it is a red flag that maybe the baby is too big to pass through the pelvis or that something is holding it back. This is one of the biggest reasons today for C-sections. For second timers, babies don't usually drop into the pelvis until

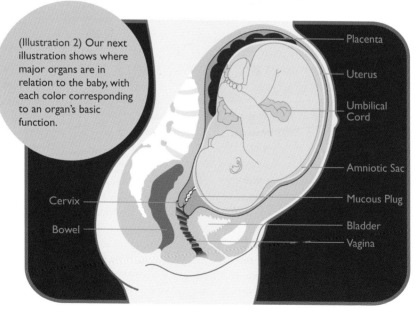

(Illustration 2) Our next illustration shows where major organs are in relation to the baby, with each color corresponding to an organ's basic function.

Placenta

Uterus

Umbilical Cord

Amniotic Sac

Mucous Plug

Cervix

Bladder

Bowel

Vagina

you are in actual labor. If the baby drops in before 36 weeks, it is a sign that the baby is possibly going to come early. So you better start packing your bags!

Our previous illustration shows where major organs are in relation to the baby, with each color corresponding to an organ's basic function. For example the yellow area is the *bladder*. Ok ladies, ask your partner if they know why it's yellow. I've asked that question in my classes at least a million times and you would be amazed with the answers I get. Even when I make it easy by telling the men that they, too, have one, I still get answers like "the fallopian tube?" As you can see from the illustration, the baby is sitting on top of the bladder. This is the reason the average pregnant mom goes to the bathroom what feels like 45,000 times a day and straight through the night. I once had a mom in my class who bitterly complained that her husband never acknowledged her many trips to the bathroom during the night. So one night she decided to climb over her husband on the way out of bed. As the woman straddled her husband's waist, he said excitedly, "What are we doing here? SEX??" Every woman in the world knows that sex was not on this pregnant mom-to-be's mind at five in the morning with a full bladder. She responded loudly, "I'm going to the bathroom ONE MORE TIME TONIGHT!!!"

Daytime peeing is no picnic either. How many of you find yourselves getting up from the toilet to wash your hands, only to discover, "Gosh I need to pee again!" That baby just loves to sit on the bladder. So for all you husbands and partners out there, acknowledging your wife or partner's bathroom visits goes a long way to making her feel like she's not alone.

The pink area is the *vagina*. It is elastic and streeeeetches beyond your wildest imagination. Thank goodness! The brown area is the *bowel*, which is also located in the same general area as the *uterus*, which is the area in dark pink. The uterus is a muscle that stretches all the way around the baby. The lowest part of the uterus is called the *cervix*. As you will see, everything is interconnected when it's time to push the baby out.

Cervical Effacement

The job of labor is to change the *cervix* in two ways. The first is to thin it out. Think about it like this. You're having a party and you need to blow up six balloons. What do you do before you blow them up?

You stretch them out, because the thinner the rubber, the faster it opens. So the thinner the cervix, the faster it opens. Unlike a balloon, however, there's nothing you can physically do to make a cervix thin. It happens naturally as part of the labor process beginning around 36 weeks. This thinning is called effacement and is measured as a percentage. Most cervices begin "LTC" - (no this is not a sandwich) which means long, thick and closed. As the cervix shortens, 50 percent means the cervix is halfway thinned and at 100 percent, the cervix is paper thin. The degree of effacement is a factor in the speed of labor. As a rule of thumb, the more effaced the cervix is before going into labor, the faster the labor.

Cervical Dilation

The second way the cervix changes is by opening up, or dilating. If we look at Illustration 3 (Cervical dilation chart), we can see what the cervix looks like dilated from one to ten centimeters. Yes, I know, it looks just like a diaphragm chart the gynecologist shows you before your fitting, but this is how the cervix dilates. Now, how is the opening measured? During an examination, the doctor uses her fingers to measure the degree of dilation. If

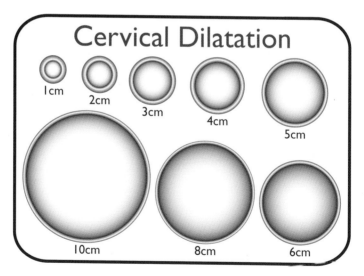

(Illustration 3) When the cervix goes from one to five centimeters, it's easy to measure with the two fingers. However, from six to ten centimeters, the cervix resembles a circle surrounding the baby's head that just continues to get bigger and bigger.

one finger can be placed inside the cervix, then the mom is one centimeter dilated, two fingers, two centimeters, etc. Contrary to popular belief, however, the doctor doesn't keep adding fingers to measure the cervix. Medical professionals are very experienced at this and can easily gauge cervical dilation.

When the cervix goes from one to five centimeters, it's easy to measure with the two fingers. However, from six to ten centimeters, the cervix resembles a circle surrounding the baby's head that just continues to get bigger and bigger. When the doctor or midwife can start to feel the soft spots on the baby's head, which are called fontanels, the cervix is dilated in the range of seven to eight centimeters. At nine centimeters, we call that a "rim," the cervix is just barely hanging on around the baby's head. At ten centimeters the cervix is considered fully dilated and the head comes through and moves into the vagina. To be clear, ten centimeters is not often the exact circumference of your baby's head, but it is a reference point for the moms. It is sometimes the case that the bigger the baby, the longer it takes for the cervix to go around the baby's head. It is also true that some labor and deliveries can be shorter for smaller babies. So now you know why your friends that delivered smaller babies had shorter labors.

As you can see from the diagram, the lip of the cervix continues to thin out as it becomes increasingly dilated. To make it clear, only until a woman is fully effaced can she dilate past five centimeters. For some moms, the thinning out process will take place while you are dilating. For others, the cervix will be completely effaced prior to going into labor and having your first labor contraction. Once again for you second timers, it will be different. With your second baby, the dilation often takes place first, followed by effacement. But as stated earlier, you will not dilate past five centimeters if you have not effaced fully. A former student, a doctor's wife, was walking around at four centimeters with her second pregnancy. She was waiting to go into labor or break her water, after which she would certainly deliver quickly. Which is exactly what happened. She broke her water and one hour later her son was born! Now that's what I call a perfect second delivery!

The Mucous Plug, Amniotic Sac and Placenta

Inside the cervix there is a *plug of mucous* (small white area in the illustration 2) that protects your baby against infection while in the uterus. The *amniotic sac* (light blue area) that surrounds the baby is a huge balloon of water, also designed to protect the baby. If you get an elbow in the tummy while riding the subway, bus, or walking through a crowded mall, you may get a black and blue mark, but the baby will feel only a little wave of water. The *placenta*, the hot pink area above, is usually located at the top of the uterus. It provides the baby with oxygen and nutrients - everything that the baby needs to grow and survive - through the *umbilical cord* that ends where the baby's belly button will be. There isn't a class I teach where someone doesn't ask me how the baby breathes underwater. A baby's lungs do not work until after they are born. Until that time, they get what they need through the umbilical cord.

You may have heard of placenta previa. It is a condition when the placenta is located below the baby's head blocking the opening of the cervix. During the 20th week, most moms have a sonogram to see where the placenta is so that there won't be any surprises down the road. If your doctor tells you that you have a complete previa, you may be placed on modified bed rest and a cesarean delivery will be in your future.

SIX PRELIMINARY SIGNS OF LABOR

So now that you have a good idea about what the body looks like from the inside and how things are supposed to work, let's talk about the next thing on your journey. In the last weeks before a woman gives birth, her body lets her know that things are getting ready for labor. These are called the Six Preliminary Signs of Labor. These preliminary signs usually happen from about five months to two weeks before labor really begins so no need to call your doctor just yet.

1. Braxton-Hicks Contractions
The first preliminary sign of labor are Braxton-Hicks contractions, which are described as practice contractions because they give you a little preview of what is to come. They usually occur around your 25th week of pregnancy and continue throughout pregnancy. Although a husband in one of my classes kept calling

these contractions "Toni Braxton" contractions, I want to ensure everyone that there is no music involved with this natural process! Braxton-Hicks contractions feel like a tightening around the belly and usually last less than 30 seconds. They can be painless or feel like a menstrual cramp or a backache. During these contractions, the uterus is tightening and then relaxing. However, near the end of the pregnancy, they come more often and can be confused with real labor contractions, which is why they are often called "false labor".

The best way to tell whether the contractions you are experiencing are Braxton-Hicks or real labor contractions is to change your activity. For example, if you are lying down, get up and walk around. If you are walking, sit down for a few minutes. If the contractions stop, you are having Braxton-Hicks contractions. Real labor contractions continue no matter what you do. So in the middle of the night when your wife is pointing to her belly with very wide eyes and telling you that she has never felt them like this before, you say, "Remember what Sheri told us to do… get up and walk around. If they stop you are not in labor." In fact, get up and walk with her. If it stops, go back to bed. You're going to need the sleep. If it doesn't, it's the real thing and skip to the next chapter right away!

2. Weight Stabilization

The second preliminary sign of labor is very exciting. You will notice it at your doctor's office a couple of weeks before labor. When I was pregnant, my doctor's nurse used to direct me to the scale and tell me to just strip from the waist down. I was taking off my earrings, my rings. I wasn't stepping on that scale with an extra ounce of weight on me! Then with much trepidation I looked at the scale with surprise only to ask her if she had changed scales on me. When she asked me why, I whispered, "I lost a pound!" YIPEE!!! Weight stabilization occurs when your body has gained enough weight, hopefully somewhere between 25-35 pounds, depending on your build.

(Illustration 4)
Weight stabilization occurs when your body has gained enough weight, hopefully somewhere between 25-35 pounds, depending on your build.

3. Burst of Energy

This will come as a big surprise after a very tiring third trimester. Once again about two weeks before labor begins, you will experience a burst of energy unheard of since you first became pregnant. Bursts of energy looks like this: your husband or partner comes home to find that the living room looks different, because you've moved the furniture around the room! Or, you may have cleaned the house from top to bottom or cooked a five-course meal. The burst of energy is your body telling you it's time to get organized and prepare for the baby, similar to a mother bird building a nest before having chicks.

The best story I've ever heard on this subject goes like this. Tom and Linda, a couple from my class, go to bed around 9 PM and Linda falls fast asleep while Tom reads a book. At 11 PM, Linda sits up suddenly wide-eyed. Tom asks if everything is all right, which Linda says yes. She heads to the bathroom and then heads down to the kitchen. As always, it's better to pee first and then have your snack. Tom thinks that Linda is downstairs preparing a little midnight snack, until he hears her on the telephone. After she hangs up the phone, he hears clinking and clanging. Now getting a little nervous, he yells down, "Honey, what are you doing in the kitchen?" Linda replies, "I decided to fix the dishwasher. I called the GE 24-hour hotline and they told me how to do it. Do you want to come down and help me?" The moral of the story: If you find yourself fixing dishwashers at 3 AM, you know you're having a burst of energy.

4. Lightening or Engagement

The fourth preliminary sign of labor is lightening or engagement which occurs when the baby drops into the pelvis and moves from floating in the -4 pelvic station (see illustration of pelvic station on page 20) down to the -3, -2 or -1 stations. In some cases, your co-workers will notice this right away and you will be able to tell by how your clothes fit. For those who are carrying your babies right under your boobs, you will notice you'll be breathing easier. You may also consider moving into the bathroom because the baby has now moved INTO the bladder. You might as well take the TV, telephone and refrigerator with you because you'll be living there full time.

Lightening or engagement happens anywhere from 36 weeks and on. If it happens earlier it may mean the baby is coming sooner. If it doesn't happen at all, the baby may be too big to pass through the pelvic bones and you should discuss this with your doctor.

5. Increased Vaginal Discharge

As a labor nurse, this was an interesting sign. When moms-to-be would come to the hospital in labor, they would often look around, check that no one was listening, wave me over and whisper, "I'm having some vaginal discharge I'm a little concerned about." I, of course, answered in my normal tone, "Don't worry about it, you are having a baby today!" And then she would shush me and repeat in a whisper, "But I'm having A LOT of vaginal discharge -- is this normal?" I had no idea where she was going with this until she finally whispered while pointing towards the door, "Is this an infection? Because if I have an infection, my husband is going to be in A LOT of trouble!!!"

Increased vaginal discharge occurs about two weeks before you go into labor and means the vagina is sending out more secretions in preparation for labor and delivery.

Most of the Six Preliminary Signs of Labor occur about 2 weeks before labor begins.

6. Diarrhea

Often the day or night before moms go into labor, they experience some diarrhea. For those of you who experienced a bit of constipation during your pregnancy, believe me this will come as a HUGE RELIEF! No doubt, you will be thrilled to share this information with your partner, exclaiming, "Honey, I've had six bowel movements today – it's been the best day of my life!" However, if you have been regular, you may be wondering what you ate to cause the diarrhea. At this stage, frequent bowel movements are a sign that the body is cleaning itself out in preparation for childbirth and usually a big tip-off that labor may start within 24 hours.

Review

After 36 weeks, the three most important pieces of information your doctor or midwife will discuss with you concern:

1) Pelvic station
2) Cervical dilation
3) Cervical effacement

Now you know when your doctor or midwife says in labor: "You're 100%, -2 and 3," you now know that means that you're 100% effaced, the baby is at -2 station, and you're 3 centimeters dilated. Also translated as: "It's a good beginning and keep up the good work! You're making progress!"

I find the Six Preliminary Signs of Labor come in real handy when your partner travels for a living. When you see four of the six signs, it's probably time to stop traveling.

Chapter Two

Sit Down, Note Time, Call Doctor, Green Means Go!

— Sheri Bayles

Three Actual
Signs of Labor
and
Two Breathing
Techniques

30-45
sec.

There are only three signs that labor has actually started. These are the big ones, the ones you really have to look for. These are the signs that tell you that the big day has finally arrived. They do not occur in any particular order - any of these signs could be your first, second or third sign of labor. Generally, we look for two signs before we call it labor.

1. Loss of the Mucous Plug

One concrete signs of labor is the loss of the mucous plug - which we all recall from the last chapter is located inside the cervix and protects your baby against infection while it is in the uterus.

How do you know when you've lost the mucous plug? Simple. When you "find" the mucous plug! And how do you find the mucous plug? Picture this. You're in the bathroom and after you've urinated something sort of drops out of you. You're not exactly sure what it is. You get brave, take a wipe, look at it and say, "What's this?" The way I describe it to you moms-to-be is that it is a white plug of mucous with a red to pink tinge to it. The way I describe it to your partners is that it looks like nothing you've ever seen before in your lives." At this point in class, the partners ask, "But how do you know that I'm actually going to see it?" Well guess who gets called first to the bathroom when one discovers the mucous plug?

Here's how it might go:

Mom-to-be: "Honey, can you come to bathroom, please. I have something to show you."

Husband/Partner (with a feeling of dread): "It's not the mucous plug is it? Because you promised me in class I wouldn't have to see it."

Mom-to-be: "GET IN HERE, I need a second opinion."

Husband/Partner (after shuffling slowly to the bathroom and looking at what she's holding): "Sheri was right. This is nothing I've ever seen before in my life! This must be the mucous plug."

Why do we call this an actual sign of labor? Well, if you look in a medical dictionary, the definition of labor is cervical change. In order for the mucous plug to drop out, the cervix had to have opened, and therefore changed. However, by itself, the loss of the mucous plug does NOT mean you are in labor. In fact the loss of the mucous plug can happen two days to two weeks before you see another actual sign. So you will not need to do anything - except throw it away. No need to save it or bronze it or dry it out for the baby's book. We trust you when you tell us you've lost your mucous plug. If this is your only sign of labor, however, you do not need to notify your doctor immediately, but inform her at your next office visit. It's also possible that you will miss this sign of labor. Don't worry – it is very common.

I am frequently asked if the baby is still protected after the plug drops out. Although the word "plug" implies that it is a plug to the amniotic sac, it is in fact a separate entity. So even after you lose it, the baby is still sitting in the protective bag of water. This is very important for those of you carrying multiples. If you see the mucous plug before 36 weeks, please call your doctor right away. This means your cervix has opened.

2. Rupturing the Membranes: Your Water Breaks

Another actual sign of labor is when the amniotic sac breaks. Also referred to as "breaking your bag of water," it can happen in two ways. The first one is known as "The Gush". Imagine yourselves walking down the cereal aisle of your favorite grocery store. You pick up a box, check the price and mutter, "Oh my! $4.50 for this?" Suddenly you stop - you feel a champagne cork pop inside you. Then a stream of fluid runs down your legs, into your shoes and onto the floor. In other words, you find yourself standing in a puddle. Naturally you think, "Oh, my gosh, I just broke my water in the supermarket! How do I get out of here without anybody noticing?" If this happens to you, consider what my former student did when this exact thing happened to her. She grabbed a bottle of apple juice and broke it right next to the puddle, pretending she had apple juice on her leg as she quickly left the store. "Clean up on aisle six!" Of course, your "Gush" could be less dramatic, but let me assure you it will always take you by surprise!

There is a second scenario that might occur. Rather than a gush, some women experience what is called a high leak, which is more of an ongoing trickle. This happens when a tiny rupture occurs near the top of the amniotic sac. It's harder to identify and you might think that it's urine or vaginal discharge. Although it sounds a bit disgusting, the best way to tell what is trickling down your leg is to smell it. Vaginal discharge has an odor, urine has both a color and an odor, but only amniotic fluid has neither a color nor an odor.

I was once teaching this to a couple privately in their home. When I told them they might have to sniff the fluid, the wife turned to her husband with a very serious expression and said, "Phil, you're going to have to sniff that for me. My nose has been all stuffed up with the pregnancy." You should have seen his face. I thought he was going to fall off the couch!

As soon as you notice that your water has broken, either by way of a "Gush" or an ongoing trickle, there are four things you have to do. It's what someone once called my mantra: "Sit down, note the time, call the doctor and if the fluid is green, head to the hospital." Now, let me explain why I'm asking you to do these four things.

1. Sit Down

Some women, especially those having their second or third baby, may have a floating baby that hasn't moved down into their pelvis. In these cases, if you stay on your feet for a long time after your water breaks, there is a chance your baby's cord might prolapse. A prolapsed cord is an umbilical cord that slips down in front of the baby's head, preventing it from being born vaginally and requiring an emergency C-section. When the water breaks the baby's head should move down, sit on the cervix and create a cork so that the rest of the fluid in the amniotic sac stays around the baby. Keep in mind that when your water breaks, it's not one gush and you're finished. It's one gush followed by lots of little gushes. So be prepared. You don't want to find yourself in some public place with water leaking out of you and all you have is a couple of tissues in your purse. Case in point. One evening I was on duty at the hospital when a woman came walking in wearing a long black flowing dress with a white towel hiked up between her legs. When I asked her what had happened, she told me that she had broken her water in a restaurant and all they could give her was a white towel. So I recommend keeping a folded up maxi pad with you when you go out.

When I say sit down, it doesn't mean that you have to sit down, put your feet up and stay there until you're allowed to go to the hospital. What I do mean is you shouldn't walk all over town. You can walk around the house, make phone calls, pack your bags and do everything else you need to do, within reason, before delivering your baby. You can take a shower. However, some doctors prefer that you <u>not take a bath</u> because they believe sitting in a body of water after your water breaks increases the chance of infection.

I want you to know this way of thinking doesn't exist everywhere. After all some women around the world deliver their babies in large bathtubs. So if you want to spend some time in the tub during labor, please check with your caregiver on what their views are on the subject.

2. Note Time
The second thing I want you to do is note the time. The reason why we note the time is because the risk of infection greatly increases 24 hours after the water breaks. Some hospitals and birthing centers want to make sure that the baby is delivered within 24 hours of the water breaking, while others feel comfortable waiting up to 48 hours and sometimes longer. Once you are in the hospital or birthing center, everyone you meet will ask you what time you broke your water. Where I worked there are five layers of staff and everyone asks every single woman in labor the same question. So many people ask, that it starts to feel like the cleaning staff mopping your floor is going to ask what time you broke your water.

For some women breaking your water, like in the case of a high leak, may not be that obvious. One of my girlfriends called me one morning and asked me if she had broken her water. She described it as soaking her mini pad in a couple of hours. I thought that was the best description.

3. Call Doctor
The third thing I want you to do is call your doctor or midwife and tell them what time you broke your water. Their first question will be, "what color is the fluid?" Clear fluid is normal, but green indicates that meconium, the baby's first bowel movement, is present (see

details in number four, below). If the fluid is clear, your caregiver will then ask if you are having contractions. If you aren't, then most likely you will be told to go about your business. Sometimes it can take Mother Nature six to twelve hours to kick in with contractions after the membranes rupture, which means you still have lots of time before any medical intervention, such as an induction would need to take place. One of the toughest things to hear from your physician at two in the morning after you have informed them of your broken clear fluid is to go back to bed. "GO BACK TO BED??? ARE YOU KIDDING?? I'M LEAKING ALL OVER MY KITCHEN FLOOR. NEXT THING I'LL BE DOING IS LEAKING ALL OVER MY BED!!" Once again be prepared. I have recommended for years to place a baby's waterproof crib pad underneath the mom-to-be's side of the bed to prevent amniotic fluid from seeping into the mattress.

4. Green Means Go!

Meconium-stained fluid looks like pea soup, in consistency as well as in color. When the fluid is green, there are usually three reasons for it: One, the baby is past its due date; two, the baby is in a breech position; or three, the baby is in distress, which means that the baby's heart rate goes down. If your baby swallows meconium he can have difficulty breathing after deliverly. The doctor will give you instructions at this point.

When I talk about meconium in class, the best way to remember what to do is, think of a traffic light: "Green Means Go". Green fluid means that you go directly to the hospital so that your doctor can check to see how the baby's doing. Green fluid isn't an emergency. It's simply a sign to go to the hospital to make sure everything's alright. You do not need to go to the closest hospital. You should make your way to your doctor's hospital. If you can't get your doctor directly on the telephone, leave a message with the service that your water is green and that you will meet them at the hospital. Don't panic - simply go.

Another thing I want you to do if the amniotic fluid is green is to feel if the baby is moving. And the best way to get the baby to move is to poke or gently shake the belly. Put your hand on your belly and push in steadily on the baby's body and the baby will react by kicking back. If the baby moves, the baby is ok. My favorite saying is: "fetal movement = fetal well-being."

Two other tried-and-true methods to getting a baby to move is drinking something cold and sweet or doing some slow chest breathing. Women also comment that babies move a lot when they lie down. When I was pregnant, my favorite time to feel my babies was in the evening when I would lay down to watch TV or read a book. My husband always called it his "entertainment", watching our boys move around inside. The way they were kicking, I could have sworn they were playing soccer every evening.

Once you get to the hospital, the staff will examine you and connect you with a fetal monitor to make sure the baby is okay. If the baby is in distress, most likely you will need to have an emergency C-section. However, if everything's normal, the odds are good that you'll have a perfectly fine labor and delivery.

Just so you know, it is not uncommon for meconium to be present in the amniotic fluid. It happens quite often. Once again, if it happens to you, do not panic. Try to get the baby to move and head to the hospital.

If you are nervous about this issue at any time near the end of your pregnancy, do not hesitate to speak with your doctor or midwife about your concerns.

A mantra to memorize when your water breaks:

1. Sit Down

2. Note Time

3. Call Doctor

4. Green Means Go! (to the hospital)

3. Contractions

This is the most common way of going into labor. But before we delve deeply into the subject of contractions, let me start by saying that real labor never happens like it does on television. So don't use soap operas, sitcoms or made-for-TV movies as your labor coach. On TV the nurses run around screaming, "They're coming every five minutes, doctor! They're coming every five minutes, doctor!" as they rush the woman into the delivery room. But in real life, when the contractions are coming every five minutes, you're at the very beginning of labor, not at the end. So when it happens to you, chill out, don't stress out!

When it comes to contractions, there are three different patterns that coincide with three different phases of labor: *early*, *active* and *transition*. First, what does a contraction feel like? The best description of a contraction is that it feels like a wave. It starts off slowly increasing gradually, hits a peak at the top of the contraction (the most painful part) and then comes down and decreases in strength to the end.

We don't care how long they last or how much down time you have. All we care about is how often they are coming from start to start. When you have had twelve consecutive contractions

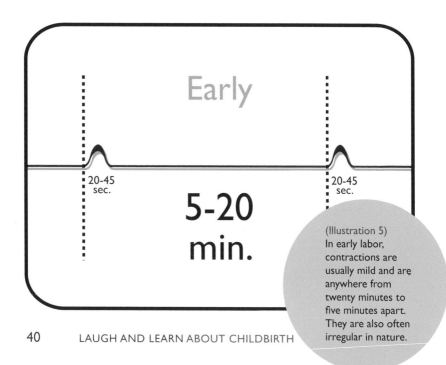

Early

20-45 sec.

20-45 sec.

5-20 min.

(Illustration 5)
In early labor, contractions are usually mild and are anywhere from twenty minutes to five minutes apart. They are also often irregular in nature.

LAUGH AND LEARN ABOUT CHILDBIRTH

that are five minutes apart, which would take an hour, pick up the phone and call your doctor or midwife.

For those of you who do not live close to the hospital, I know you're thinking, "We're not going to wait that long. There's no way we're waiting that long. If we wait that long, we won't make it to the hospital in time." Well, unless your doctor or midwife tells you to get in the car and get moving, resist the urge to rush! Believe me you will get there in time, probably too early, as a matter of fact!

Many times a doctor or midwife will talk with you on the phone about how you are feeling in order to decide whether you are ready to come to the hospital. Here are two likely scenarios: Your water hasn't broken yet and the contractions are coming every five minutes. You're thinking, "Oh my, I'm in labor! This is it!" You pick up the phone to call the doctor.

First scenario:

"Hi Dr. So-and-so. Yes. Uh-huh, I'm contracting every five minutes. I was told to call you now. Yes, it's kind of exciting. No, not that painful. The weather outside? Why are you asking me about the weather outside? I just told you I'm in labor!" This is when your doctor starts chatting because she wants to know how you are doing with the contractions and whether or not you can talk through them. "No my mother-in-law doesn't live in town. No, we're not very close anyway. Uh-huh, so listen, I'm having a contraction right now. Yes! Like a menstrual cramp, very reasonable. But listen, I'm a little nervous. It's our first baby and I really would like to come to the hospital. No? Not yet? When's yet? You don't know? So you want me to call you when the contractions get stronger? When I CAN'T TALK through the contractions? HOW AM I SUPPOSED TO CALL YOU IF I CAN'T TALK THROUGH THE CONTRACTION?? All right, all right. I understand. I'll call you then."

Second scenario:

"Hi, Dr. So-and-so. Yes, I'm having contractions every five minutes. Yes, they're kind of getting stronger now. Yeah! They're ... there're getting really hard now!! Uh-huh, I'm having one! ... I'm having one right now! ... (HEAVY BREATHING) ... you want me ... (HEAVY BREATHING) ... I'll be there in 15 minutes."

The Big clue for the doctor:
If you can't talk through a contraction, you're in labor!

In order for labor to work, it has to be painful. I know that's not what you want to hear, but as they say in the gym "no pain, no gain." And that's exactly the truth of labor. If you can still smile and laugh during a contraction, you are NOT in labor. If you CAN'T talk during a contraction, you ARE in labor. Which is why you are the one the doctor has to speak with, not the partner, friend, or mother. The doctor wants to gauge your condition directly.

Some doctors aren't that good about keeping you on the phone and they just say, "Oh, every five minutes, come on in." But you don't have to rush. You still have plenty of time.

Let's review before moving on:

THREE ACTUAL SIGNS OF LABOR

1. Loss of Mucous Plug
If this is your only sign of labor, you do not need to notify your doctor immediately but inform her at your next office visit, that is if you haven't yet experienced any other actual signs of labor. It's also possible that you will miss this sign of labor. Don't worry. This is very common.

2. Membranes (Water) Breaks

Follow the mantra: Sit down, note time, call doctor, green means go (to the hospital).

3. Contractions

If contractions have started before the membranes (water) break, which is the most common scenario, call the doctor when contractions are five minutes apart as measured from the start of one contraction to the start of the next contraction.

BREATHING TECHNIQUES

Lamaze breathing has changed from its inception. For many years Lamaze taught three breathing techniques that went along with the three phases of labor. Well, as the organization has grown, it has continually updated and changed. What we noticed over the years was that most women used the first breathing technique, but then abandoned the breathing to either other comfort measures or medication. To understand what the breathing does for you, let me give you a little introduction.

Whether you choose to take pain medication or not, learning the Lamaze breathing techniques will help you tremendously through early labor. When labor gets stronger, you can make the decision about getting more help to cope with the pain. First, let me give you a little background on how these breathing techniques came to be.

As I said in the Introduction, back in the 1950's, a French obstetrician named Dr. Lamaze discovered that women could handle the process of labor without being completely anesthetized if they could focus their attention on something other than the pain. He found that if you give a woman something to do while she's in labor, breathing, relaxation techniques, staring at something on the wall, she can deal with the pain. Today this method is commonplace, but then it was revolutionary. Keep in mind that back in the 50's, 60's and even the early 1970's, women were still knocked out during labor. The whole idea of keeping a woman awake during childbirth was really avant-garde, especially in the United States.

As a mother, OB/GYN nurse and a childbirth educator, I know the

Lamaze breathing and distraction techniques really work. But Lamaze is more than just breathing, it's a philosophy that teaches that childbirth is NOT a disease - it's a normal process.

When you can control the pain of childbirth through breathing and other techniques, you are in charge of the birthing process. Rather than being a patient in a hospital at the mercy of the well-meaning medical staff, you become an empowered woman experiencing the miracle of birth. By managing your own pain to the very best of your ability, even if pain medication becomes necessary, you, your partner and new baby are the stars of the show, not the doctor, midwife or nurses. This is the way it should be.

First Breathing Technique: Slow Chest Breath

For you ladies, there are three rules of breathing:

1. Choose a focal point. A focal point is something you look at and don't move your eyes from, like a picture, a magazine cover, even a stuffed animal or rosary beads that you can stare at while breathing. When you're packing to go the hospital, find something that you can take with you, something that has meaning for you and you like to look at - but nothing that can break if it falls off your bed, like that priceless Ming vase, okay?

2. Take a cleansing breath. Take a cleansing breath at the beginning and end of every breathing technique. A cleansing breath is best described as a slow breath in through the nose, and a slow breath out through the mouth. You use it at the beginning and end as a signal to your partner that you are starting and ending a breathing technique. It also gives the baby a much-needed shot of oxygen for the contraction.

3. Practice in one-minute intervals. During labor, most of the contractions last a minute, so get comfortable breathing for that amount of time.

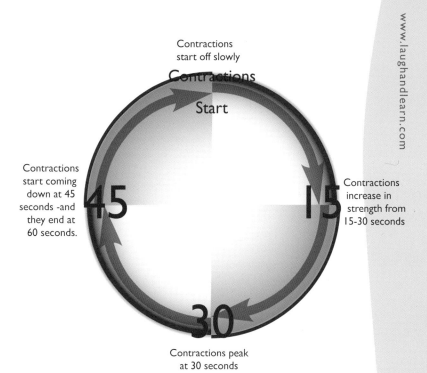

Contractions
start off slowly

Contractions

Start

Contractions
start coming
down at 45
seconds -and
they end at
60 seconds.

45

15

Contractions
increase in
strength from
15-30 seconds

30

Contractions peak
at 30 seconds

For partners, there is one rule:

Tick off the time every 15 seconds when practicing at home with the moms-to-be, because that is the way contractions work. They start off slowly and increase in strength at 15 seconds - they peak at 30 seconds - they start coming down at 45 seconds - and they end at 60 seconds.

Now let's learn the slow chest breath that is used in early labor. It is just like the cleansing breath, only slower. The normal breathing rate for an adult is about 12 to 16 breaths per minute. What you need to aim for is six to twelve breaths per minute and your partners are going to count the breaths, not including the cleansing breaths. Remember, slow breathing doesn't mean holding your breath. We just want to keep the breathing nice and slow. Also, the breaths don't have to be very deep, that can be difficult with a baby sitting right under your lungs. The goal is to control the rate of the breathing, not the depth of the breath.

Here are the steps to take when practicing (which I suggest doing one minute a night):

Moms, first find a focal point and concentrate on looking only at that object. Take your first deep cleansing breath and blow that out. Follow with your slow chest breaths, breathing very slowly in through the nose and out through the mouth. You may find it helpful to slowly count to yourself five seconds while inhaling and five seconds while exhaling.

Coaches, count the number of breaths silently in a one-minute interval while marking off the 15 second intervals out loud.

At 60 seconds you will end by taking another deep cleansing breath.

Don't worry if you don't get it perfectly the first time. Keep practicing until you get the rhythm of it by slowing down and concentrating on your focal point. If you can't breathe in through your nose due to allergies or other reasons, it's okay. Breathe in through the mouth and out through the mouth. Just take it as slow as you can.

Begin using this technique when you can no longer walk, talk or joke through a contraction. This technique takes your attention away from the pain by focusing on your breathing. Does it take away all the pain? No. I can tell you from personal experience that you will still feel your contractions. When I was in labor, people I worked with would come in and visit me while I was breathing. As a Lamaze instructor at the hospital where I gave birth, I was under a lot of pressure to perform. I felt like a monkey in a zoo. But even despite those less than optimal conditions, the breathing techniques actually worked for me. I still felt the pain, but the choice was either scream or breath. And my decision to breath was the better way to stay in control. The choice to breathe is yours. You don't have to resort to the medication immediately because there are ramifications if you take the drugs too soon. This breathing technique helps you to get a little bit further into your labor before you make the choice about pain medication.

Second Breathing Technique: The Hee-Hee's

This breathing technique has been taken out of our renewed curriculum because most women didn't like it and very rarely used it. We also found that most women would just change the rhythm of the first technique to suit their needs instead of using this technique. We have left this in the book for those Lamaze purists. However if you find this one too hard to do, don't panic. Just use the first one and change the pace to make it work.

The second breathing technique is affectionately called the "hee-hee's" because that's what it sounds like when you're doing it. It is a short, shallow pant. You take the air in through the mouth and out through the mouth. When exhaling say "hee" gently. Make sure to breathe evenly in and out. If you don't, you might send out more air than you're taking in and begin to hyperventilate. If you start to feel light headed, slow down. When you slow down your breathing, you'll notice that you will get more breaths in which will correct whatever funny feelings you're having. Just a slight warning for partners: When the mom-to-be begins this breathing, this is the phase of labor when she's most likely to grab you by the collar and yell, "BREATHE WITH ME!" So do it. Okay?

When you practice the "hee-hee's" the same breathing rules apply:

Pick a focal point.

Take in a cleansing breath.

Begin the "hee-hee" breathing technique.

Practice for one full minute.

Take one last cleansing breath at the end.

Practice this every night for one minute also and you'll be ready for the big day.

The great thing about the "hee-hee" breathing technique is that we can prove that it works before labor happens. Do this experiment:

Partners: Place your hand on the mom-to-be's thigh and squeeze her thigh like a contraction squeezes the uterus. Watching the clock, you will begin the contraction. At five seconds, you will begin to squeeze her leg increasing the strength of the squeeze every 10 seconds until you reach the 25 second mark. From 25 to 35 seconds hold the hardest part of the squeeze. From 35 to 45 seconds lighten the grip. From 45 to 55 seconds lighten it more. At 60 seconds stop completely. I know you don't want to do this, but squeeze hard - really hard (no bruising please). Don't go too easy because even as hard as you can squeeze you won't be able to get close to how painful a real contraction is.

Moms-to-be: No matter what happens, breath using the "hee-hee" breathing technique until your partner's hand comes off your leg. Do not look at your leg and do not look at your partner. Keep your eyes on your focal point. Then take a cleansing breath.

To prove that it works, partners, squeeze her thigh as hard as you did at the peak of the simulated contraction. If you've both done our little experiment properly, what you moms will find is that the pain caused by the second leg squeeze was much worse than the pain you experienced during the time you were breathing and concentrating on your focal point. In fact, the difference in the level of sensation can be huge. Let me explain why. Our brain can only pick up on one stimulus at a time. If there is more than one stimulus, the brain will pick up on the one that is closest to it. When you're concentrating on breathing, you are so busy with trying to do it right that you don't feel the pain coming up from the uterus nearly as intensely. And to make it work even more effectively, the partners should do the breathing right along with the moms during labor. It really helps the concentration immensely, which is why it really pays for both the partner and the moms-to-be to practice this technique until you both can do it easily.

Now that we all know how to do it, at what point in labor do we begin breathing like this? The answer is simple. Start the "hee-hee's" when the slow chest breathing stops working. How do you know the first one stopped working? Because the pain is more intense. It's best to keep using the slow chest breathing as long as you can, because it's easier to maintain than the "hee-hee's."

The "hee-hee's" really work and are the bridge to getting you to the time when you have to decide whether or not you want pain medication. Now, since the partners are going to be breathing with the moms during labor, they should know that this technique really works. So, let's reverse the roles in our "hee-hee" experiment. Moms-to-be act as the coaches and partners take the role of the moms-to-be. To make it more effective, moms-to-be can use two hands to make a harder squeeze. Ready! Set! Go! Now everyone is almost ready for the big day.

My favorite "hee-hee" story, or "don't go to the hospital until you're ready to bite off your toes!"

A wonderful couple, Janice and Phil, started me off on my third year of teaching Lamaze classes. At the time, my office was located right next to the admitting labor room where they stopped first on their way to delivering their baby.

Phil knocks on my door at around thee o'clock in the afternoon.

"We're here," smiles Phil, "I'm so glad you're here, too!"

I smiled back and asked if Janice was in labor.

"Yes, she's contracting every five minutes just like you said."

Phil then pulls out a yellow legal pad, on which he has listed EVERY contraction for the last three hours.

"That's impressive," I said. "How is Janice feeling?"

"She feels great," Phil replied.

Uh oh, I think to myself. "If she's feeling great she shouldn't be here yet, Phil."

"No, no, Sheri, I'm telling you, she's in labor!"

We walk down the hall together and there is Janice sitting on the bench. "Hi! Sheri, I'm here. I'm in labor. I'm so glad!"

"Janice", I said, "you're not in labor."

"Yes I am. I really am! My contractions are coming every five minutes just like you said!

"No, Janice. You're supposed to call your doctor when your contractions are coming every five minutes, not come to the hospital!

"But Sheri, I'm really in labor!"

"Janice, I want to tell you something, once they examine you, you are going to be sent home. Why? Because you look too good."

She's then taken in to be examined. She's two centimeters dilated

CHAPTER TWO: THREE ACTUAL SIGNS OF LABOR   49 and contracting every five minutes. A perfect labor. But it's just the beginning. So they send her home. Before leaving Phil pops his head into my office one more time.

"Sheri, remind me again when we're supposed to come in."

"Simple. When Janice is ready to bite her toes off."

Five hours later I'm teaching a class, and there's a little knock on the door. Phil pokes his head in.

"Sheri, we're back, and Janice is NOT HAPPY."

I excuse myself from the class and walk into the hallway where I see Janice very slowly walking toward me moaning, "heeee......heeeee......heeee" in a most pitiful way.

"NOW you're in labor, Janice! Go get examined."

Janice was seven centimeters dilated so they took her to the labor and delivery unit. One hour later she was fully dilated and she had her baby without medication, which was a total surprise to her — and a great testament to the power of the hee-hee's.

Lamaze breathing techniques
are just one tool of
many comfort measures that
you can use in labor.

Chapter Three

The question I get asked most about is
"How will I know I'm in labor?"

— Sheri Bayles

Labor:
Stage One

In this chapter you will learn everything there is to know about labor and delivery. But to begin, I would first like to give you the six care practices that will help you achieve a normal birth:

The Six Care Practices:

1. Labor SHOULD happen on its own.
2. Women SHOULD have total freedom of movement in labor.
3. Women SHOULD have continuous support during labor.
4. NO routine interventions during labor.
5. Women SHOULD NOT give birth on their backs.
6. Mother and baby SHOULD NOT be separated after birth.

Each of these care practices will be discussed in detail during the next couple of chapters.

The question I get asked most about labor is "How will I know I'm in labor? Will I recognize it from the beginning?" Don't worry. You will eventually recognize it. But at the beginning, when the contractions start, they may resemble menstrual cramps, backaches, or even Braxton-Hicks contractions, not what you would consider real labor pains. Relax. You will eventually figure out that you are in real labor. The information in this chapter will help you, and always remember your doctor is only a phone call away. I can almost guarantee that you won't be standing in your living room, pointing to a baby on the floor and saying, "DID ANYONE SEE WHAT HAPPENED HERE?!"

As you may have noticed there have been a lot of trilogies in discussing childbirth. Labor is no different. It takes place in three stages.

Women should have continuous support during labor.

Stage One: The period when the cervix opens from one to ten centimeters.
Stage Two: The baby is born.
Stage Three: The placenta or after birth comes out.

LABOR: STAGE ONE

Stage One is the longest stage and is subdivided into three phases: (1) the early phase; (2) the active phase; and (3) the transitional phase. Within each phase, something different occurs.

Early Phase
In the early phase of labor, the cervix opens from one to three centimeters, the contractions begin coming anywhere between 5 to 20 minutes apart from start to start, and each contraction lasts only 30 to 45 seconds.

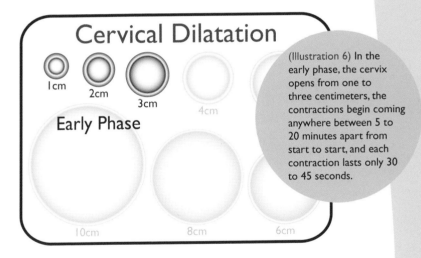

Cervical Dilatation

1cm 2cm 3cm 4cm

Early Phase

10cm 8cm 6cm

(Illustration 6) In the early phase, the cervix opens from one to three centimeters, the contractions begin coming anywhere between 5 to 20 minutes apart from start to start, and each contraction lasts only 30 to 45 seconds.

Don't start timing contractions until they begin to hurt.
Most labors start with an irregular pattern, so assuming you have not ruptured your membranes, i.e., broken your water, how do you know you're in labor? Well, you don't right away. So, if you think you're in the early phase of labor, don't start timing your contractions until they begin hurting. Why? Because it can be quite some time before they are painful so you might as well relax until then. When the contractions begin to take your breath away, begin timing them.

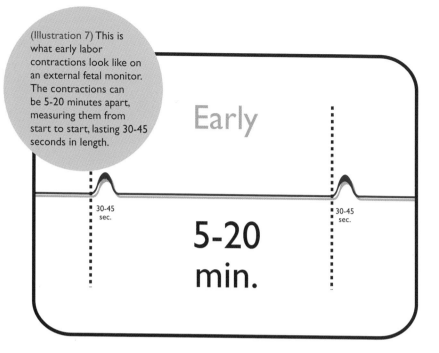

(Illustration 7) This is what early labor contractions look like on an external fetal monitor. The contractions can be 5-20 minutes apart, measuring them from start to start, lasting 30-45 seconds in length.

Early

30-45
sec.

30-45
sec.

5-20
min.

When the contractions start hurting, stop eating solid foods.

In birthing centers and more progressive hospitals, you may be allowed to keep eating during labor, but most hospitals only allow clear liquids during labor. Tea, broth, Jell-O, soda or juice, anything you can pour into a glass, hold up to the light and see through, is a clear liquid. The reason we put you on a clear liquid diet in this phase is because during this phase you feel fine, but during the next phase, you might start feeling nauseous. So if you decide to eat pancakes and sausage during the early phase of labor, we're all going to see it again in the next phase when you bring it back up. Partners, your clear liquids are gin, vodka, beer, and wine. Just kidding! There's still a long way to go, and you'll need to be sober. Trust me on that one!

Entertain yourselves.

My next suggestion in the early phase of labor is entertain yourselves. Moms, you're going to feel great, both emotionally and physically. You begin to realize, "I'm having a baby!" Your partner might be surprised at how good you look during this period. This is the phase when labor hurts the least and since it can take 10-12 hours until the contractions begin coming every five minutes, you need to fill the time and keep busy. So, rent a video, get your nails done, go shopping, take a shower. Distract yourself!

But don't do what a patient of mine did during labor. She and her husband went to the movies to pass the time and decided to see a lengthy foreign film with subtitles. For three hours the woman kept thinking, "I'm in labor, and I'm sitting here reading subtitles. Can this get any more surreal?" Do yourselves a favor and rent a video to view at home. It's a lot cheaper and you can stop and start it at any time.

Partners, this is the phase when the mom-to-be needs you the least. So take advantage and use this time to get yourselves organized. When the contractions are coming every ten minutes, you have an hour to two hours to get your act together. When they get to five minutes, get yourself home as fast as possible, if you're not there already! During this first phase of early labor, take the time to eat something, but DON'T do it in front of your wife! It's not fair for her if you're sucking down a roast beef sandwich while she's eating Jell-O, okay? I once saw a husband waltz into labor and delivery with some fast-food french fries from McDonalds. Let me tell you, that incident did not go over well.

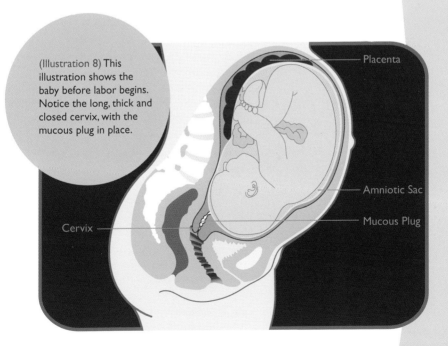

(Illustration 8) This illustration shows the baby before labor begins. Notice the long, thick and closed cervix, with the mucous plug in place.

Placenta

Amniotic Sac

Mucous Plug

Cervix

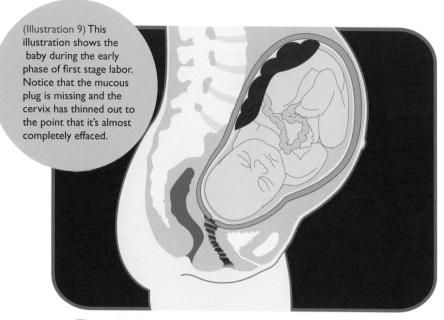

(Illustration 9) This illustration shows the baby during the early phase of first stage labor. Notice that the mucous plug is missing and the cervix has thinned out to the point that it's almost completely effaced.

The early phase of stage one labor takes the most time and is the least painful. When your contractions begin coming every five minutes, you pick up the phone and call your doctor. She will decide whether you should stay at home, go to the hospital, or make a trip to the office for an examination. When you get examined, the doctor will determine how many centimeters dilated you are, how effaced you are, and the station of the baby. If you are between one to three centimeters dilated, often your doctor will tell you to take a walk for about an hour or two. When you return, depending on how much progress you have made, they will either decide to admit you or possibly send you home. By the way, walking is a great way to help the cervix open and move the labor process along. You can walk outdoors or in the corridors of the hospital, whatever suits you.

Another little warning is in order for partners. At first, the walk may go fine. The moms are doing the slow chest breathing and feeling just fine. After a while however, things might start to change. The moms will begin walking a bit slower, the looks on their faces will change as the pain from the contractions increases. And then it starts: The moms may begin to whine. Now if you have never heard your wives whine before, this may be a shock for you. But it is really a good sign because it means your beautiful wife is moving into the active phase of first stage labor.

Active Phase

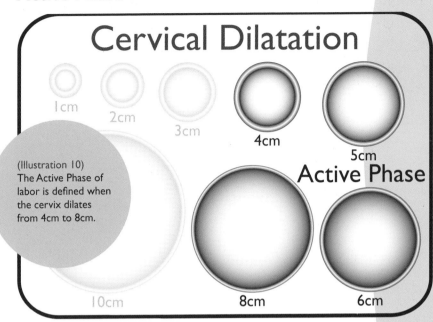

Cervical Dilatation

1cm
2cm
3cm
4cm
5cm

Active Phase

10cm
8cm
6cm

(Illustration 10)
The Active Phase of labor is defined when the cervix dilates from 4cm to 8cm.

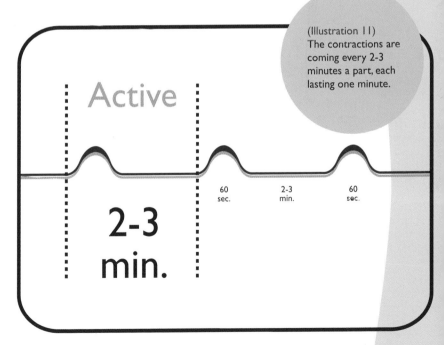

(Illustration 11)
The contractions are coming every 2-3 minutes a part, each lasting one minute.

Active

60 sec.
2-3 min.
60 sec.

2-3 min.

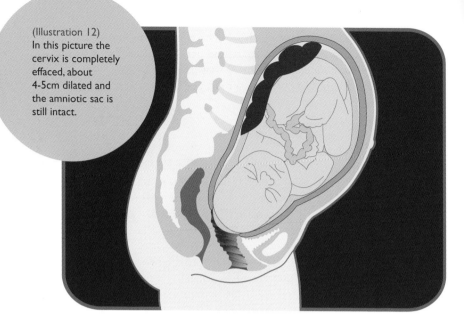

(Illustration 12) In this picture the cervix is completely effaced, about 4-5cm dilated and the amniotic sac is still intact.

A second clue that your wife is entering the active phase of labor is when she begins making no sense whatsoever when speaking. Here's a conversation that I overheard recently as one of my couples was entering active labor:

Woman: Let's go home now. We can have the baby tomorrow.

Man: Honey, you're in labor and you're four centimeters dilated. We can't go home now. What's the problem?

Woman: I don't know. I just think it would be nice if we had the baby tomorrow. After all, it is your father's birthday. It would be a nice gesture.

Whether your wife gets a bit irrational or not, most women are admitted to the hospital during the active phase. It lasts from four to six hours on average and begins when the cervix opens from four centimeters all the way to eight centimeters. The contractions are coming every two to three minutes apart from start to start with each contraction lasting one minute.

This means that the mom-to-be has one to two minutes between contractions without pain to relax and get geared up for the next one. The difficulty of labor is that as it progresses, the contractions get longer but the intervals between contractions get shorter.

Hydration

Many women, once admitted to the hospital, have IV's inserted to keep hydrated. Not all hospitals or all doctors do this, but many do. Dehydration can bring on fever in the mother, which then means that the babies have to be tested for bacteria after birth. It just makes sense to try to avoid that scenario, if possible. Sipping clear liquids can also help avoid this. In some places, a "heparin lock" may be available. This is when a small IV hub is placed in your arm for later use and you do not need to be hooked up at this time. The less intervention at this point, the better. You will also have much more mobility without an IV.

Rupturing the Membranes Manually

For you moms who haven't ruptured your membranes spontaneously, this is the time that some doctors choose to rupture them manually. They do this with an instrument called an "amnihook" that looks like a crochet needle. It seems scary, but it's a painless puncture. The amnihook doesn't hurt when it goes into the vagina. In fact, the procedure feels like an internal exam. The doctor breaks the water and the water in front of the baby's head comes out.

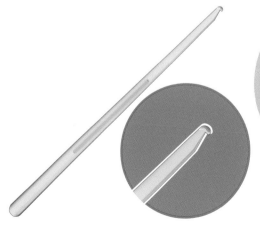

(Illustration 13) This illustration depicts the amnihook, which is used to manually rupture the amniotic sac (bag of water).

In my experience, it is best not to break the water artificially unless there is a medical reason. We have learned over the years, that the amniotic sac is a wonderful cushion for the baby. It also takes the pressure off the cervix for the mother. If a mom is laboring well, breaking her water will only make it more difficult and painful. In most labors, it is a totally unnecessary procedure. In my opinion, there are only two medical reasons to rupture someone's membranes manually. One is when the baby's heart rate is showing signs of distress and the doctor needs to see if there is meconium in the fluid. The other reason is to help progress a very slow or stalled labor. However, if you get up and move around, your labor will start progressing on its own.

I advise that you discuss this possibility with your doctor beforehand and let them know that you would prefer not having it done unless there is a valid medical reason.

Back Pain in Labor

One in five women experiences back pain in labor. In the past, it was believed that this was caused by the baby's position in the pelvis. Normally, the baby faces the mom's spine as it descends into the pelvis. Every once in a while, a baby faces the side. Sometimes, the baby faces up in what we call the "sunnyside up" position.

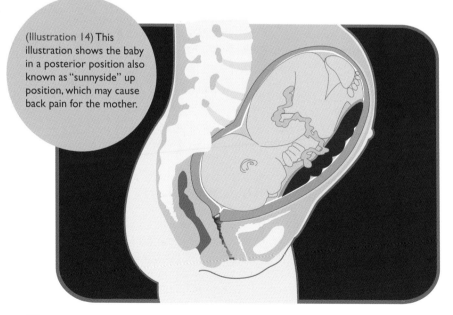

(Illustration 14) This illustration shows the baby in a posterior position also known as "sunnyside" up position, which may cause back pain for the mother.

In this position, the back of the baby's head has direct contact with the mom's spine with every contraction. Needless to say, this particular position makes labor even more painful than with a frontal labor. However recently we have discovered that women can experience back pain in labor even when the baby is in the right position. Unfortunately, we usually don't know who will experience back pain until it happens in the active phase.

(Illustration 15) If you do experience back pain, the worst position is to lie on your back. My advice is try lying on your side or sitting over the back of a chair and have your partner apply counter pressure by pushing on the small of your back with his hands during a contraction.

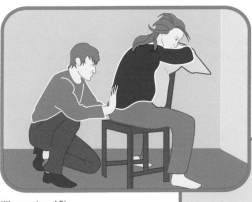

(Illustration 15)

(Illustration 16)

(Illustration 16) Another option is to position yourself on all fours, which takes the pressure off the spine. In this position, your partner can also perform a double hip squeeze by placing one hand on each of your hips and squeezing in simultaneously. Many women feel great relief with this technique.

Walking around can also help with the discomfort as can sitting on a birthing ball. (Illustration 17) In the hospital, we sometimes put the bed all the way up and hang the mom-to-be over the back of the bed. I know it sounds like preparation for some medieval torture, but it is actually a great position to alleviate the back pain of labor. (Comfort Measures on page 66) After hearing about back pain in labor, every pregnant woman wants to know about epidurals and pain medication. I will discuss this completely in chapter five. Just so

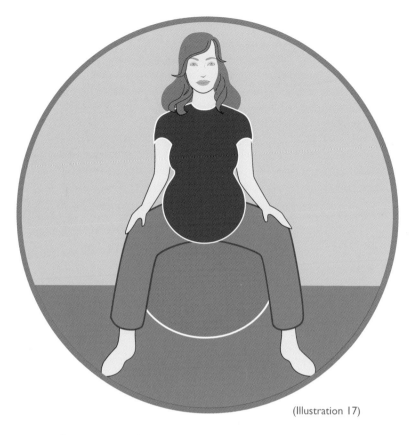

(Illustration 17)

you know, pain medication/epidural is usually administered during the active phase of labor and takes all the pain away.

Bloody Show

Another thing that may happen during this phase of labor is bloody show, which is a continuation of the mucous plug, but a little more bloody with a little more mucous. Yes, it can be described as icky, icky, icky. When women experience this at home, many of them head straight to the hospital. Do not be alarmed if this happens, bloody show is not a hemorrhage; there won't be a lot of blood on the floor. It's a little bloody mucous and it means that as the cervix is opening, some capillaries are breaking in the process. The blood mixes with vaginal discharge and creates the bloody show. It is very common and nothing to be alarmed about.

Modesty

Just so you partners know in advance, a woman in labor can get very hot. Your beautiful wife begins her hospital stay by lying on the bed with a little gown on, a sheet over her, and maybe two little monitor belts. By the end of active labor, the sheet is gone, and most likely even the gown. Now she's naked and all of a sudden a medical student walks in and says, "Hi! I'm here to draw your blood." Partners do their best to cover their laboring wife, but wives generally don't care at all. Let me tell you from experience that labor gets a woman in touch with her body more than any other event, and I have to warn you that it doesn't stop with the birth of the baby.

In addition to being an OB/GYN nurse and Lamaze instructor, I'm also a Lactation Consultant. I once went to visit a new mother to see how she was getting along with breast feeding and wasn't surprised to find her sitting on the bed naked, except for a pair of bikini undies, breastfeeding her new baby. In the baby business, this is a common sight, so I wasn't shocked until I looked around the room and saw a man sitting in the corner. Once I realized it wasn't her husband, my new mother turned and said, "Oh, Sheri! I'm sorry, I didn't introduce you to my father-in-law, Joseph." I turned every color of the rainbow, but he just sat there reading The New York Times. The great thing about newborn babies is that their arrival makes the most unlikely scenarios seem absolutely normal.

Nausea and Vomiting

As if the pain isn't enough, sometimes nausea and vomiting accompany active labor. As unpleasant as it is, the good news is that it won't last forever and the baby is on his way! I have found in my experience, that sucking on an ice pop may help alleviate the nausea.

Comfort measures used in labor include birthing balls, hydrotherapy and positioning of the mother.

Comfort Measures

The beginning of active labor is where partners come in. You will probably be called upon to offer emotional support or comfort. The moms-to-be need you to get them water, juice or ice chips, rub their legs or back, or anything else that is humanly possible for you to do. Remember to have patience, lots of patience, because there are several phases to your job.

The next phase might be called the "Jekyll and Hyde". Your wife may want you to provide comfort measures, but she's not convinced that they'll work. She'll ask you to rub her legs. You will. You'll ask her if it's helping. She'll yell, "NO, get your hands off my legs!" You'll feel helpless and useless, but your job's not over yet, not by a long shot. Next she'll grab you by the collar and scream, "BREATHE WITH ME!" But you won't be doing it right. So she might throw you out of the room and you'll happily skip to the door. But wait! You hear a little voice in your head, it is my voice, and it says: "NEVER leave your wife in active labor." Do you know why? Because this act of abandonment will come back in every fight you have for the next 25 years and you don't want to be discussing this when your child is graduating from college! All kidding aside, being the partner is a difficult job, but always remember, you're not the one in pain. So just hang in there, do the best you can, and everything will be all right. Of course, there are lots of women who are completely civil to their partners and the above scenario may never take place. You just being there is often all the support she will need.

Hydrotherapy

Hydrotherapy is considered one of the best comfort measures for a laboring mom. Standing or sitting in a shower, helps women deal with the pain of labor beautifully. After all, when does a shower not feel wonderful? In my earlier nursing days, I watched many a midwife move a mom- to-be into the shower when she was four centimeters, only to come out an hour or two later a full eight to nine centimeters. Showers help relax a mom which in turn lets the uterus contract more effectively.

In some progressive hospitals as well as birthing centers, there are also Jacuzzi tubs that women sit in during labor. In fact in some places around the world, women deliver their babies in bathtubs. Feeling buoyant and surrounded in warm water is a soothing and wonderful way to pass the time of labor. If you are thinking about using hydrotherapy, my advice is to find out ahead of time if your facility has showers or tubs that you may use while in labor.

Birthing Ball

Another comfort measure used often in labor is the birthing ball, sometimes called exercise balls in gyms. Sitting on a birthing ball widens the pelvis and allows the baby to descend properly. You might also feel more comfortable sitting on something with a little give. Let your partner help you onto the birthing ball and stay close to help with your balance.

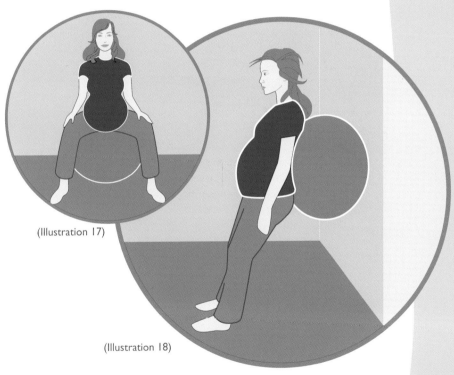

(Illustration 17)

(Illustration 18)

Birthing balls can also be placed against the wall (see illustration 18) and you can lean into it with your back. Spread your legs a little wider than shoulder width and you will be able to lunge from side to side, which also helps with the baby's descent.

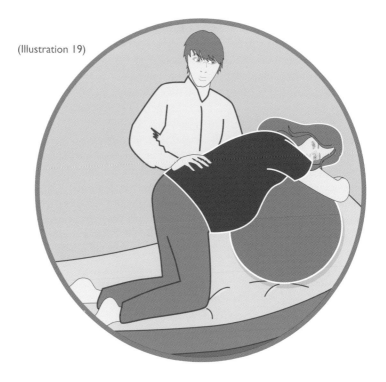

(Illustration 19)

And the third use is hanging over the birthing ball on the bed. The pressure of the ball on the abdomen can help move the baby down. (Illustration 19) Other uses are seen in the following illustrations.

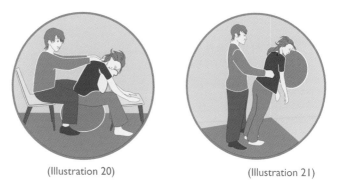

(Illustration 20)   (Illustration 21)

Mothers in labor enjoy sitting on the birthing ball with their partner behind them massaging their shoulders. (Illustration 20) Another use of the birthing ball is to place it against the wall at shoulder height, lean in on it with your husband applying pressure to your back or hips. (Illustration 21)

Many birthing facilities may have a birthing ball on hand, but my advice is to buy one ahead of time, so you can also use it at home when labor begins. You can then carry it in with you and use it at your hospital or birthing center. When you buy it, make sure it is big enough for you so you are actually sitting on it instead of squatting. My only other advice is to buy the air pump with it. It makes blowing up the ball so much easier ... for your partner. You will find having the birthing ball around after you deliver will help you get back into shape faster. They are great to do sit-ups on. You can find the birthing ball and pump at my Web site, www.laughandlearn.com. Please note that it is important to find the right size birthing ball depending on your height.

Hiring a Doula

In addition to the above comfort measures, I strongly advise thinking about hiring a labor doula. In the research, it has been proven that having a doula with you helps shorten the labor and also avoids the likelihood of a cesarean section. A doula is not a doctor, midwife or nurse. She is a trained professional whose job is to provide physical and emotional support for you during the entire birthing process. Hiring someone who is specifically trained to provide support can take a lot of pressure off your partner, who may not feel completely comfortable in the role. I have found that the best way to find a labor doula is to ask your childbirth educator or doctor for a referral, or contact the Doula Organization of North America at (888) 788-3662 or online at www.dona.org.

Hiring a labor doula often ensures a better outcome with your labor and delivery.

Heat and Cold

Alternating hot and cold temperatures can help alleviate pain. A hot water bottle placed on the abdomen and/or back can be very comforting, as are warm or hot towels placed on the perineum (the area around the vagina). Cold compresses or cold packs can help numb pain. Warm lavender rice socks can also help. Many labor doulas use these in their practice.

Rice Socks:

Fill a new mens' tube sock or knee sock ¾ full with uncooked white rice. Add dried lavender or a few drops of lavender oil to the rice. Tie a ribbon or string tightly around the top, or sew closed. Heat the sock in the microwave one to two minutes. Shake the rice around to make sure the heat is evenly distributed. Place on the body where relief is needed.

The sock can also be chilled in the freezer to make a cold pack.

Vocalizing

Some women find it very helpful to moan or groan during labor. Releasing pent up emotions through vocalization can be a great way to stay centered and focused. But beware many hospitals frown upon vocalization. To be honest, it makes many staff members nervous and uncomfortable when they hear someone moaning or grunting. However this is your labor and my advice is to do whatever works for you.

Transition Phase

We've finally reached the last phase of the first stage of labor: transition. And just when you think it's bad, it gets worse. This phase takes place when the cervix opens from eight to ten centimeters. It's the last two large circles highlighted in the Dilatation Chart (illustration 22, below). At this point, the contractions are coming every 60 to 90 seconds and they last 60 to 90 seconds, which

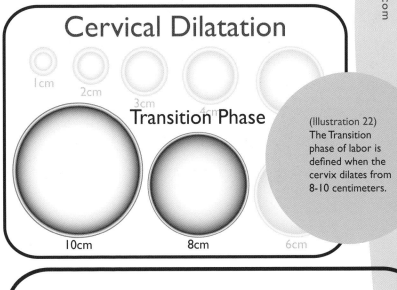

Cervical Dilatation

1cm
2cm
3cm
4cm

Transition Phase

10cm
8cm
6cm

(Illustration 22) The Transition phase of labor is defined when the cervix dilates from 8-10 centimeters.

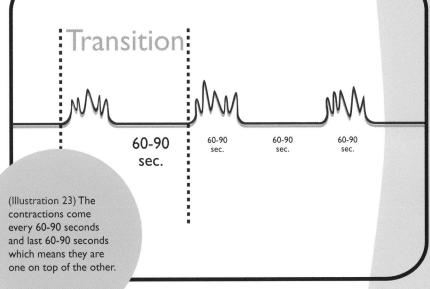

Transition

60-90 sec.

60-90 sec.
60-90 sec.
60-90 sec.

(Illustration 23) The contractions come every 60-90 seconds and last 60-90 seconds which means they are one on top of the other.

means that they are coming one right after the other with no break in between. The bad news is that it's the most difficult phase of labor, but the good news is that it's the shortest, lasting only one to two hours.

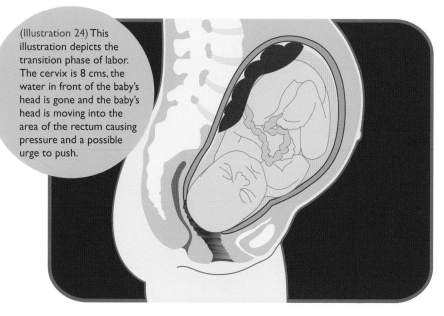

(Illustration 24) This illustration depicts the transition phase of labor. The cervix is 8 cms, the water in front of the baby's head is gone and the baby's head is moving into the area of the rectum causing pressure and a possible urge to push.

During this phase of labor, your baby's head begins pushing on the rectum, which makes you want to bear down and push. But if you begin pushing too soon, you'll push the baby into the cervix and doing so in that manner could make the cervix swell up and begin to close. Similar to when one gets punched into the eye, and the eye swells and closes up. In that circumstance, your cervix, which had dilated to eight centimeters, might go back down to six centimeters and stay that way, ultimately necessitating a C-section.

To avoid this scenario, your nurse or midwife will be watching you very carefully at this point so that you don't ruin your labor. After all, you've come so far! They'll keep you from pushing too soon by telling you to open your mouth and blow. Imagine a whole bunch of candles sitting on top of a birthday cake, and blowing out each candle individually.

It is impossible to blow out through your mouth and bear down at the same time, so this technique really works. Mary, one of my clients, had a very fast labor. She was at home when her labor started and the pain seemed manageable. After a little while, Mary decided to take a shower and wait for her husband to come home. When the shower was over, the pain was so strong that she couldn't get out of the tub. Her husband, Bob, who was home by now, helped her out and then took her to the doctor's office. At first the doctor wasn't too concerned because it was her first baby. But when she examined her, she was shocked to discover that she was already nine centimeters dilated. They jumped in a cab. All the way to the hospital while Mary screamed, "I have to push the baby out!" Her husband yelled, "Blow those candles out! Blow those candles out!" Just so you know, the breathing worked and she gave birth to a beautiful baby in the hospital in record time. They are still grateful that it didn't happen in the cab.

Usually when you feel the urge to push, the doctor will examine you to see how dilated you are. If you do get an epidural prior to this phase, you will not feel this urge to push. Instead, you will feel rectal pressure because the baby's head is moving down.

When you reach ten centimeters, you'll get the green light to push. Now the fun really begins! When my doctor gave me the news, I truly wanted to get off the bed and click my heels in the air, because I knew that it wouldn't be long before I saw my new babies!

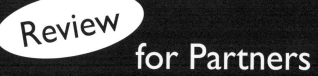

Review for Partners

Early Phase: Take care of your own business so that you'll be emotionally and physically available to your wife.

Active Phase: Embrace your role as the comfort measure person and do your wife's bidding to the best of your ability.

Transition Phase: Be there. Aloha! Enjoy the ride!

To be honest, during the transition phase, there's not much you'll be able to do to help your wife. I often advise not to say much to your wife at this point, but ahhh … you men love a challenge. Some of the statements I've heard come out of partners' mouths: "You look beautiful!" which of course is not true since your wife is sweating bullets. Or, "If I could take the pain away from you, I would!" Yeah, right! Liar, liar, pants on fire! (And your wife knows you are lying through your teeth.)

Try as you might, in this case less is more. All the loving words in the world don't work in this moment. Pain does that to a person. A woman has to be incredibly focused to deliver a baby without an epidural. Don't take anything personally and you'll be in good shape.

Here is my favorite partner story: Once upon a time, not too long ago, I walked into the birthing room to check on one of my patients. I was surprised, to put it mildly, when I found the partner parked between his wife's legs at the foot of the bed shouting into her vagina: "Look for the light now! Aim for the light!" I asked him what he was doing and he told me he was giving his child directions. Needless to say, while strange and funny, this technique doesn't work.

Transition is the hardest but shortest phase of labor.

Chapter 4

The NEW way of pushing is totally geared to what the mother feels. This is called spontaneous pushing.

— Sheri Bayles

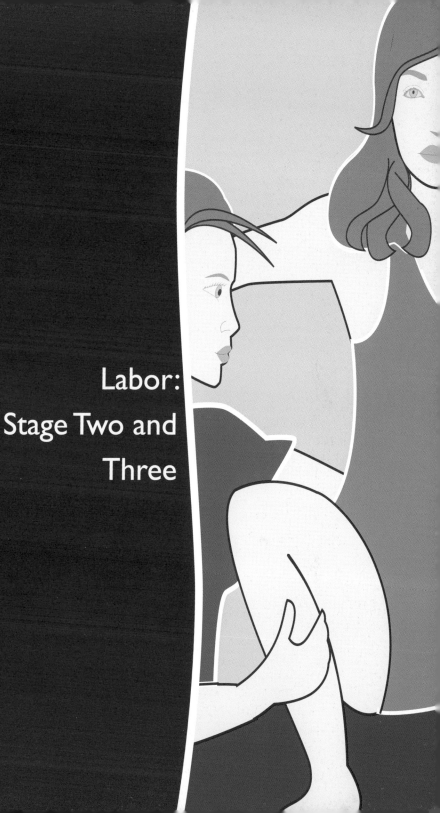

Labor:

Stage Two and

Three

The second stage of labor begins when you start pushing. One of my favorite questions to the partners in my class is, "So, how long do you think it takes to push a baby out, from the time the mom-to-be is fully dilated to the time you see the top of the head?" I love the answers I get. Most of the partners will tell me anywhere from 5 minutes to 30 minutes to 6 hours. At this point, I then ask them to picture themselves in the bathroom with a watermelon in their rectum and ask how long it would take to push that out? The expressions on their faces are priceless!!

They are always surprised when they hear it takes one to two hours to push a first baby out. The difficulty is in the exhaustion level of the mom-to-be at this point. She may have labored ten to twelve hours (not uncommon for first labors) only to be staring at one to two more hours of pushing, which can be a lot of work. But the good news is that labor slows down and the contractions lighten up.

Episiotomy

Bigger babies, eight pounds or over, need more room than smaller babies and the mother can tear in the process. As the baby's head starts to appear, the decision about whether the doctor should perform an episiotomy needs to be made. An episiotomy is a small cut in the perineum, the area between the vagina and the anus, to facilitate the birth of the baby.

When I first began working in this field, it was rare to see someone not get an episiotomy. But as times have changed and we're understanding more about the process of birth, it has been determined that in many cases, episiotomies are often unnecessary. In fact for most women, the tear that may occur is often less problematic than an actual cut to that area. Also the tear is more natural, thus the healing is often less painful than an episiotomy.

However, every doctor looks at episiotomies differently. Some are more eager to cut than others, and midwifes are usually more conservative, resisting the procedure unless absolutely necessary. It is important to discuss this subject with your caregiver before the day of delivery. In fact I usually recommend bringing it up in the last weeks of pregnancy, so you can get a feel for what your caregiver believes. It also doesn't hurt to let them know that you would prefer not to have one unless absolutely necessary. If you avoid an episiotomy during your delivery, you will be sitting on your rear end a whole lot easier following your delivery.

Pushing

Pushing for some women can be difficult, especially for first timers. For others it may be a breeze. One huge factor is whether or not you have had an epidural. If you have had an epidural, you may have lots of energy, but may have a tough time getting your muscles to work right. You will be numb from the waist down but you should feel rectal pressure. You can also use a mirror in labor so that you'll be able to gage your progress by watching the baby's head descend.

If you haven't had an epidural, you may be exhausted, and yet for some of you, the hardest part of the process has arrived. While many mothers comment on how good it feels to push when they have the urge, others may be very tired. My analogy to pushing is as follows: You have trained to run the New York City marathon. You are emotionally and physically ready to handle the challenge. The big day arrives and you have run the 26.2 miles to the end. You get over the finish line only to find out that you have an additional half-mile to run. That's pushing! In other words, you get to ten centimeters and you think you are done but now the hard part starts – getting your baby out. You tell yourself that millions of women have done it, and you can, too. You muster up reserves of energy and strength you didn't know you had, and you do it. That was my story, and that will be yours. The good news is that in one or two hours (sometimes much less for you second timers) you'll be holding your baby in your arms.

Positions

Squatting

The best position for pushing your baby out is a squat. If you haven't had an epidural, you'll have control over your legs and will be able to get into this position. The use of a squatting bar is most helpful now along with the support of your partner or nurse on either side of you. (Illustration 25, next page) Most of us aren't used to squatting so it can be a bit uncomfortable, but since you'll have gravity working for you, it's the most effective position.

Squatting widens the pelvis 40 percent more than the next best position and can really speed up the process. If you want to practice squatting in order to get in shape for labor, you can squat down, place a pillow between the upper and lower parts of your legs (behind your knees) to take the pressure off your thighs. Then follow the breathing/pushing technique outlined below while in this position. Keep in mind that if you are hooked up to a fetal monitor, it can sometimes be impossible to squat. In that case, get yourself into the position where you are sitting up as much as possible.

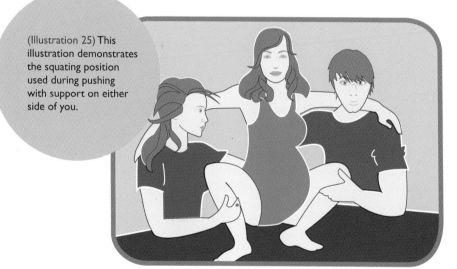

(Illustration 25) This illustration demonstrates the squating position used during pushing with support on either side of you.

Second stage of labor begins when you start pushing your baby out.

Modified Sitting Up Position

Due to extensive epidural use, this is probably the most common position used in hospitals. (Illustration 26) With an epidural, you won't have complete control over your legs so your best bet is the modified sitting up position. You can practice this position by sitting on your bed or on the floor with one or two bed pillows between your back and the head of the bed or couch.

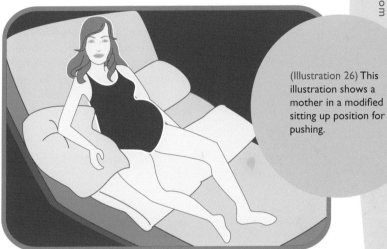

(Illustration 26) This illustration shows a mother in a modified sitting up position for pushing.

Next, put the soles of your feet together, letting your legs flop to their sides on the floor/bed. If you put the soles of your feet flat on the bed or floor, your pelvis closes up, which inhibits the pushing process. Pull your legs slightly out which will widen your pelvis more and you are good to go. On a birthing bed, there are footrests that will help support your legs. An old technique that is still being practiced today is to have a nurse on one side and a partner on the other side holding the mothers' knees up near her ears. Not only is that incredibly uncomfortable for the mom-to-be but it also it stretches the ligaments beyond what is normal. It is believed that when a mother's legs are stretched that far back, the vagina will shorten. In my experience, it does not help at all but only makes the mom sore the next day and may damage muscles. Again, insist on leaving your legs where they are comfortable.

Technique

Only through practice will you get a feel for pushing, and the more you practice, the more prepared you will be. Make it a habit: Practice one minute a night until you go into labor. If you are activity restricted, please check with your doctor to make sure you are allowed to practice.

By the time you start pushing, the contractions will last one minute – which is when you push — then you'll have a break for three to five minutes. In recent years, the technique for pushing your baby out has become more user-friendly. For many years, the way we taught women to push was called "directed pushing". This way of pushing had the mothers hold their breath for ten seconds at a time while pushing down and repeating this a few times during the contraction. Well, as in all things, with research we found that this is not the most effective nor safest way to push your baby out. When you hold your breath for ten seconds, you are not only cutting off the oxygen to your body, you are also affecting the baby's oxygen supply, which in turn brings the baby's heart rate down. At that point, the staff may overreact and before you know it they are pulling out forceps or a vacuum, or discussing the possibility of a Cesarean (C-section).

As a Lamaze instructor, we are constantly updating our teaching techniques, but that doesn't always apply to a hospital staff. If you have a nurse who has worked in labor and delivery for 20 years and she feels she knows what's best, you may face some resistance to anything new.

The NEW way of pushing is totally geared to what the mother feels. If you are fully dilated and have the urge to push, you should follow that urge with small easy pushes (pushing down like a bowel movement), lasting only a second or two and repeat as often as comfortable. This is called "spontaneous pushing". You should NOT hold your breath, but rather breathe through the contraction, similar to lifting weights at a gym.

If you do not have an urge, you should wait for it to come. This way, the baby will also have a chance to "labor down". This is a term we use when the contraction of the uterus does the work and pushes the baby into the vagina on its own. This way of pushing is so much easier for the mother and less exhausting. It is also better for the baby. For moms who have had an epidural, however, this pushing may be more difficult. The lack of feeling in your bottom may make it that much harder to feel the urge to push. In that case, I recommend you let the epidural wear off slowly, so that you can feel pressure. You do not need to let it completely wear off because the pain may be way too distracting. However, if you have rectal pressure during the pushing phase, it will be much easier to follow what your body is telling you to do.

When I teach pushing to my couples, I discuss both ways. I also advise them to negotiate with the staff if needed. For example, if the nurses start talking about holding your breath during the pushing, ask her if you may try a new way that you learned. Tell her you want to push your way for 30-40 minutes and if there are no results, you will try her method. This way you won't be putting any noses out of joint. However, if the nursing staff insists on you pushing with the directed pushing method, delay that for as long as possible so the baby has a chance to labor down and try not to hold your breath for more than five seconds during a push. Also take lots of deep breaths in between to keep the oxygen flowing to both you and the baby.

In recent classes, my couples have taken great issue with having to negotiate. Change is often a gradual process. With enough time, we may just change the way some nurses and doctors look at pushing a baby out. After all, the idea of birthing rooms was a foreign concept – if not totally radical – in most hospitals until patients started demanding them. Now they are as commonplace as epidurals.

Bowel Movements

Many women ask the same question, "If I'm pushing as if I'm having a bowel movement and there's something in my bowel, will it come out?" The answer is yes, and it is very common and no nurse, midwife or doctor cares one bit about it. In fact, we take it as a good sign because it means you are pushing correctly.

If you are concerned about this, or are easily embarrassed, consider giving yourself an enema before going to the hospital. It won't hurt the baby and may even speed up your labor. The time to do it is at the beginning of your labor when your contractions are coming every 10-15 minutes apart. It takes about 20 minutes for the enema to work, so stay in the bathroom! From the 1950's through the 1970's it was very common to give women enemas and to shave their pubic region. We don't do that anymore, so if you want an enema, follow the instructions on the package and administer it yourself. You'll feel more relaxed when you're pushing.

Practice makes perfect, so let's review the DO's and DON'T's of pushing:

DO use gravity.

DO squat if you have the strength.

DO raise the head of the bed as high as possible and add a couple of pillows behind you for support if you have had an epidural.

DO insist on leaving your legs where it is most comfortable.

DO small pushes (like a bowel movement) when the contractions arrive and you have the urge to push.

DO trust your body to know what to do.

DON'T push or give birth on your back.

Your baby will arrive soon. You can count on it.

The sequence of events in this stage of labor is to push for one minute, break for three to five minutes, and then push again for one minute. It's difficult because there are usually no quick results, but eventually, you hear someone say, "There's the head!" and you know you're in the home stretch. With the next contraction comes a little more head ... and a little more ... and a little more ... and then THE HEAD COMES OUT! At this point a most interesting thing happens. When the baby comes out, most times it is facing the floor but then rotates to the side to allow for the shoulders to pass through the pubic bone. In some places the doctor may then suction out the nose and mouth to remove any fluids that have accumulated there. With the next contraction you push for the top shoulder, then you push for the bottom shoulder, and voila, after the shoulders are delivered, the baby literally flies out! They are slippery little devils! Contrary to popular belief, we medical professionals do not hang your child upside down and smack it on its rear end right after it is born. Instead, we put the baby on your lap where they usually begin screaming. If they don't, we rub their backs or tap their feet and that usually gets them going.

Cutting the Cord

Next, we clamp the umbilical cord nearest to the baby and again nearest to the placenta and then cut the cord. This is the time when you partners get your big moment, so try to stay alert! A few years back I was visiting a couple during the delivery of their baby when I leaned over to her husband (an editor at *Parent's Magazine*) and asked him, "David, are you going to cut the cord?" He replied, "No, that's not for me." What he didn't know was that his wife's doctor had all the dads cut the cord. So when the time came, the doctor asked him to come around his wife's leg, pick up the scissors and cut the cord. Which is exactly what he did. When he came back around, I asked him, "David, do you know what you just did?" "No," he said calmly. When I told him he had just cut the cord, he shockingly replied, "No, I didn't!"

Now that's a guy who knows how to follow instructions!

APGAR Score

After the cord is cut, your baby is on its own. This is when most hospitals evaluate the baby and give him an "APGAR Score" based on five criteria:

Appearance (skin color of the baby)
Pulse
Grimace (reflex response)
Activity (movements)
Respiratory

Each criteria is rated zero, one or two, with two being the highest and best. We add all five scores together to get a final score, with ten being the highest score possible. The APGAR evaluation is done twice, once at one minute after birth and another at five minutes after birth. So the baby receives two scores.

The doctor and nurse probably won't directly inform you of the baby's APGAR score, but they might be shouting it back and forth across the room, so you'll most likely hear, "What is this baby's APGAR?" "Eight/Nine!" Any score above a six is fine. A score of five and below is a sign that the baby is not reacting properly. Two scores of five or below and the baby is transported to the intensive care unit. This scenario is most common with premature babies.

Just to make you feel a little bit better, most babies do not come out with low APGAR scores unless there have been warnings during labor and delivery. In most cases, it's when the baby's heart rate keeps dropping. Normally, however, most baby's APGAR's is above seven or eight.

I was once reading the baby announcements in the New York newspapers and someone actually put their baby's APGAR scores in the baby announcement. In case you're wondering, high APGAR scores are unlikely to help get the baby into a competitive private pre-school – so don't worry about it!

Additional Procedures

After the APGAR evaluations are done, the nurses take over and perform five different procedures. In most birthing centers, mothers and babies are not separated while these following procedures are being done, as mother and baby should not be separated after birth. My advice is you can ask your caregiver what is common practice in their facility following the delivery.

1. The baby is wiped down. Believe me, they are not pretty after their grand entrance into the world.
2. Erythromycin ointment is placed in the baby's eyes. This is actually the law in some states. When the baby passes through the vagina, it is possible to pick up bacteria, which usually goes right into their eyes. In some birthing centers, they may delay this procedure so that the mother

and baby have more time to bond.

3. An identification bracelet is placed on the baby. Obviously, the hospital wants to ensure they know the child belongs to you.

4. The baby is given a vitamin K injection. The injection is given in the thigh. Some babies are born with a deficient clotting factor. Vitamin K helps with clotting and boosts clotting ability in a newborn.

5. A copy of the baby's footprints. Footprints are given to the parents as a keepsake.

The baby is then wrapped in a receiving blanket and the cutest little hat is put on its head. Wrapping the baby up snugly in a blanket is very calming during the first four to six weeks. The bundled baby is usually then delivered to the partner because there is a third and final stage of labor to come – the delivery of the placenta.

LABOR: STAGE THREE

Between five and 15 minutes after you deliver your baby, the doctor will push on your tummy while you push in order to dislodge the placenta, which looks like a liver from the butcher shop. The most important part of this final stage of labor is for the placenta to come out in one piece, which we call "intact." If pieces of the placenta are left inside it's called "retained" and problems can result, including hemorrhaging and infection. But you don't have to be too concerned about this; if you've had a normal, healthy pregnancy there shouldn't be any problems with the placenta.

In some hospitals, mothers receive Pitocin after delivering their babies. Pitocin is the synthetic version of Oxytocin, which is a natural female hormone. It causes uterine contractions and helps to induce labor before birth, and to expel the placenta after birth.

After the placenta has been delivered, we collect a small amount of blood from the umbilical cord to check the baby's blood type and then we say "Sayonara!" to the placenta. If you are banking cord blood, this is when they will collect the stem cells.

Cord Blood Banking

Everywhere you look these days, whether it be pregnancy magazines or doctor's offices, there are materials and advertisements for banking umbilical cord blood. I would be remiss if I didn't write a little about this procedure.

Cord blood banking is the collection and freezing of a baby's umbilical cord blood stem cells. To be clear, this is not the same thing as the controversial harvesting of embryonic stem cells. Cord blood stem cells come directly from the baby's umbilical cord and there is absolutely no ethical or political controversy surrounding it. So why is this done? Though there are also some genetic diseases that can't be treated with a baby's own cord blood, at the time of the writing of this book, it has been already well established that stem cells can treat and cure more than 40 diseases including many cancers and immunodeficiencies. In addition to what these cells are already doing, there is a lot of work being done figuring out how cord blood stem cells might treat heart disease, stroke and other diseases impacting nearly every family in some way in the future.

There are two options for your baby's cord blood. One is to donate to a public bank (public banking) and the other is to save it for your family's use (family banking).

With public banking, your are donating your baby's cord blood to a general bank that has been set up in your area and works with your hospital or birthing center. It would be important to find out if this is an option in your area before making any decisions. The two limitations associated with public banking is that for some areas in the country, there are no public banks. However, there are plans for a national public bank sometime in the future. The other limitation is if you donate to a public bank, your family will not have access to that cord blood even if you should need it. You will, however, have access to the cord blood that has been donated by other families.

When you save cord blood specifically for the potential use by your family, it's called family banking. Family banking is available no matter where you live and is an option that thousands of families do every single month and is a very common procedure in hospitals around the country. With family banking, you contact the banking company before you deliver the baby. They will explain how it is done and then send you the materials you will need ahead of time. You must bring those materials with you to the hospital, so at the time of delivery, your OB will collect the umbilical cord blood. This is a completely painless and safe procedure for both mom and baby.

After your OB collects the cord blood, you contact the banking company who arranges the pick-up by a special courier service, which will come to your hospital bedside and transport the cord blood to its laboratory. It is really quite easy.

At the laboratory the company will then separate out the stem cells for freezing. (Exact details on these procedures and the collection of cord blood can be seen on my DVD *Laugh and Learn About Childbirth*)

The limitation of family banking is that the fee for banking cord blood privately can be considerable for some families. It may pay to ask around because some companies offer payment plans to help make it affordable.

Another limitation associated with family banking to keep in mind is that there is absolutely no guarantee that the umbilical cord blood will be a match for a family member or provide a cure. One significant benefit of having cord blood stored specifically for your family is that there is evidence showing that treating patients with related cord blood, which means from within the family, has a much higher success rate than cord blood used from a donated source outside the family. In addition, the cord blood collected will only be enough to treat one family member. Researchers are working on a technology to overcome this limitation by expanding the cord blood stem cells so that they could be used for multiple treatments, but this technology is not currently available. With family banking, the stem cells can be used for all family members.

Some families see cord blood banking as an insurance policy. My husband and I were talking about this the other day and the analogy he made was to automotive airbags. When they were first available, you had to pay extra. People had to think about whether or not to pay for that extra protection. Of course, no one ever thinks they will have to use them, but if you are in an accident you're certainly glad you have them. This is how I see cord blood banking. If you ever need it, you will be happy you have it. Just like airbags, I think in a few years' cord blood storage has the potential to be a standard option in healthcare.

It should be noted that the American Academy of Pediatrics has made a statement that it is unnecessary to bank your cord blood privately and that the chances that you will need it are very low. This statement should not be overlooked, but I would say that you should absolutely do your own research. Find out as much as you can about it, and then make your decision. With everything concerning your baby, you want to know about all your options, and it would be very wise to learn all you can about cord blood banking.

The Facts About Cord Blood Banking are Simple:

- Cord blood stem cells can treat and cure more than 40 known diseases.

- A lot of research is being done using cord blood stem cells to treat heart disease and stroke.

- Family cord blood has a better success rate than cord blood donated from outside your family.

- The chances of using it may be relatively low now, but the value of cord blood is increasing with new research and technology.

- Cord blood banking is a non-controversial, safe and painless procedure for both mother and baby.

- Cord blood has been proven to be viable for 15 years, and the data points to it lasting a lifetime.

Breastfeeding Immediately Following Delivery

Bonding with your child for the first time is a very emotional and magical moment. If you are breastfeeding, the nurse will help place the baby onto your breast. However, as a Lactation Consultant, I have been told by many of my moms that the baby was just too sleepy or disinterested to nurse immediately following the delivery. My advice if this happens is simple: Unwrap the baby, so you can place the baby skin-to-skin on your chest between your breasts. Be sure to keep the baby's back covered with the blanket and the hat should remain on the baby's head.

In many instances, if you do this, the baby will actually start searching for the nipple. If given this opportunity, some babies will even attach themselves to the nipple, which is astounding considering they are only minutes old!! If your baby still seems uninterested, no worries, you can try again in an hour or so. Mothers who have been on an epidural for some time often have a very sleepy baby following delivery.

As a Lactation Consultant, I cannot stress enough how important it is to start breastfeeding as soon as possible. Babies are most alert for the first two hours after delivery. If we can get the baby on the breast as early as possible during this window of time, imprinting takes place. In the animal kingdom, imprinting means that the first thing an animal learns it repeats. It's the same with babies. When a baby goes onto the breast when he is most awake and alert, he latches on, sucks, and learns that his food comes from this process.

While in the womb, babies have been sucking on their fingers, which is why their little hands are always next to their faces when they nurse. Babies, who learn right away to get their food from their mother's breast, wake up when they are hungry and know exactly what to do. The long-term benefits of breastfeeding for you and the baby have been stated over and over again in the literature, but the immediate benefits have to do with your uterus and the bleeding that takes place after delivery. When the baby starts nursing, a signal in the brain sets off a chain reaction of hormones, which causes your uterus to start contracting and bringing it back into place. This also helps decrease your bleeding that comes from the uterus after you deliver. Mothers also feel very connected with their newborns when they nurse them immediately following their delivery.

When my sons were born, I had the utmost pleasure of nursing them one at a time in the delivery room. When each of them latched on, I wanted to cry in joy. Ok, I was crying anyway when they arrived, but this was the icing on the cake. I felt so connected to them and that connection continues many years later.

If for some reason it isn't possible to get your baby on your breast within two hours after birth, it's a more difficult process. So if you plan to breastfeed, and I hope you are, please communicate your desire to your doctor and the nurses so they can make sure to accommodate you if at all possible. You can find much more information about breastfeeding on my DVD *Laugh and Learn About Breastfeeding,* which is available on my Web site www. laughandlearn.com.

While you are bonding with the baby, the medical staff will stitch you up if necessary, clean you and place an ice pack on your bottom, which can get quite swollen after pushing. There will still be some bleeding, so the nurses will give you sanitary napkins.

You will have the baby for about an hour, depending on the hospital. Then the baby will be taken to the nursery to be evaluated, bathed and weighed. Often, mother, father and child go as a unit. If you're concerned about being separated from your baby at this time, please speak with your doctor in advance to understand your hospital's procedure.

CONGRATULATIONS! We've made it this far and you now have a lot of knowledge under your belt about labor and delivery. Whatever you do, DON'T forget to take a picture of your new family after your beautiful new baby has been born! Every OB/GYN nurse in the country knows how to use any type of camera, so don't hesitate to ask them.

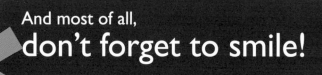

And most of all,
don't forget to smile!

Make sure to let the nurses know that you plan to breastfeed and that you want to start as soon as possible following your delivery.

Chapter 5

To avoid the cascade of interventions, it is recommended to labor as long as possible before using medications

— Sheri Bayles

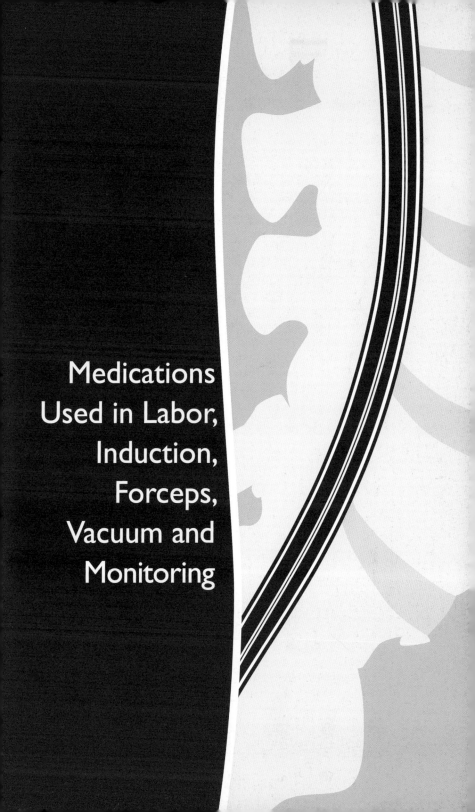

Medications Used in Labor, Induction, Forceps, Vacuum and Monitoring

As you can see from the title of this chapter, the subject matter is very medical with little laugh in it. It can also be a bit frightening. Relax. Giving birth to a child is simply an adventure into the unknown. The good news is that millions of women have gone before you and have handled all kinds of births, from the very easy to the very difficult. The other good news is that your doctor or midwife wants to do everything she can to make sure that your delivery goes as smoothly as possible. If you feel yourself getting a little nervous as you take in the information in this chapter, remember that knowledge is power. Most likely you will never need any of this but the better informed you are, the better decisions you will make should any complications arise.

If you want to give birth as naturally as possible, please make sure to speak with your doctor or midwife before you go into labor so they know your wishes. Also, make sure that your labor coach or doula is informed of your feelings on the subject. There is absolutely no reason to be timid about expressing how you would like your labor to go. It is your life and your baby. Be clear about what you need and want.

MEDICATIONS

Most hospitals will not administer pain medication until you are four centimeters dilated. Until then, you're still in the early phase of labor. The two types of pain medication available – analgesics and anesthetics – slow your labor down if administered before four centimeters, which is the beginning of active labor. That's not to say that if your labor is full blown or out of control at two centimeters that your doctor won't give it to you, it's just that from a medical point of view we want to avoid slowing down your labor as much as possible.

Analgesics

Most analgesics are narcotics like Demerol and Stadol. They are administered intravenously (IV) or intramuscularly (IM). If given IV, it is very fast acting. If given IM, it will take 10-15 minutes to feel the effect. Opposite to common belief, these drugs do not take the pain away, but help to take the edge off the contraction by raising your pain threshold, helping you to relax between contractions. But it can also make you quite groggy and a bit disoriented.

Remember, because you will feel pain, you will still need to use the comfort measures described in the previous chapters at the start of every contraction. For those of you who haven't slept too well during the last weeks of pregnancy, you might actually fall asleep between contractions, which will be a welcome relief. But let your partner know that he will have to wake you up at the beginning of the next contraction so that you'll have time to breathe through it. Otherwise, you might not wake up until the contraction peaks and the pain at that point will be extreme and very unpleasant.

The analgesic of choice is usually administered on an hourly basis when the mother is between four and eight centimeters dilated. Before four centimeters, the labor may slow down. After eight centimeters, the drug - which passes through the placenta - makes the baby groggy and sluggish, lowering his APGAR scores. It can also make you feel nauseous, which is not pleasant, especially during labor. If you are considering using an analgesic, keep in mind that once you've reached eight centimeters, you will still have an hour or two until you're fully dilated and then another hour or two to push the baby out. This drug is most effective when you are having a fast labor, which is more common for second pregnancies. For someone who is having a very slow labor, an epidural is a much better option.

Anesthetics
Epidurals are the most common drug used for labor pain, and for good reason. They are:

• Continuous (it is ongoing)
• Regional (numbing from your knees to your belly button)
• Anesthetic (which means no pain)

The pros for epidurals are:

1) There is no pain, which of course is why women love it.
2) They can be used for C-sections. When an epidural or spinal is used during a C-section, you are awake and directly involved in the process. When you are under general anesthesia, this is obviously

not the case, which is why epidurals or spinals are the first choice drug for C-sections.

In most cases the use of general anesthesia is only for emergency Cesareans when there isn't enough time to place an epidural or spinal.

But just as there are very positive aspects to having an epidural, there are also negative aspects:

The Epidural passes to the baby: It was believed for a long time that the drug didn't pass through to the placenta; however, current research suggests that it is indeed not the case. Epidurals do, in fact, pass to the babies soon after administration and there is some effect to the baby. (Especially if you have been on it for hours) We see this in their inability to organize their suck, which inevitably affects how they nurse or bottle-feed.

No walking: Because you will be numb from the waist down to the knees, you won't be able to walk. Walking is the best way, thanks to gravity, to make labor progress faster. In addition, epidurals are motor blocks so they can actually stop your uterus from working. To counter this side effect, Pitocin (see page 103) often needs to be administered to augment labor. There is such a thing as "walking epidurals," which I will discuss later in this chapter.

You'll need a catheter: The numbness makes peeing impossible. Don't worry, you won't be incontinent, you simply won't know when you have to go to the bathroom because you won't feel anything. In most cases, you'll be catheterized, either with a straight catheter, which empties the bladder and is then removed, or with a Foley catheter, which stays in the entire labor. Should you need a catheter, don't worry, you won't feel a thing thanks to the epidural.

Inability to push: Most doctors try and slow the effect of the drug down as you near the time to push so that you'll at least feel pressure on your rectum and will be able to push. If you don't feel anything at all, it is very difficult to push, especially when it's your first baby.

Blood pressure drop: When the mother's blood pressure

drops, the baby's heart rate goes down. When this happens, the medical staff quickly gets to work to bring the blood pressure back up. One method to avoid this blood pressure drop is to give two liters (2,000 cc's) of fluid intravenously prior to the epidural. If you're a person with low blood pressure or suffer from postural hypotension, meaning that you feel ill or dizzy when you get up suddenly, you might be more at risk for this. If you're a person with normal blood pressure, you probably won't have this problem.

Hot spots: Small areas, sometimes no larger than a pinpoint, that for some reason do not go numb after the epidural has taken effect. Occasionally, half the tummy area goes numb while the other half does not. In that case, we increase the dosage of epidural and that almost always does the trick.

The shakes: Shivering, shaking, and teeth chattering, thankfully lasting only around 30 minutes.

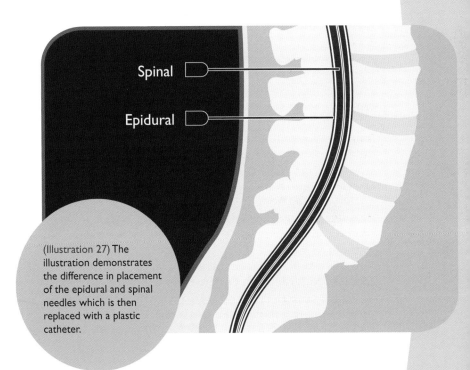

Spinal

Epidural

(Illustration 27) The illustration demonstrates the difference in placement of the epidural and spinal needles which is then replaced with a plastic catheter.

Sometimes they don't work: Usually this only happens if you had scoliosis as a child or if you have had a back injury that resulted in scarring in the spinal area. Most hospitals will try four times to make the epidural work and after that the analgesic is the only alternative.

The last issue that you need to know about epidurals is how they are administered. After cleaning and numbing your back, a rather large needle is placed in your back to get to the epidural space. As you can see from illustration 27, the epidural space exists outside the spinal column. The anesthesiologist inserts the needle outside the dura, which is a very thick membrane that covers the spinal nerves, and into the epidural space. We then replace the needle with a tiny plastic catheter that is attached to a syringe or a pump. The drug is administered through the catheter, which then bathes the nerves around your belly and takes the pain away. Additional doses can be administered every two hours through the syringe and catheter, or it may be placed on a continuous infusion pump. Each anesthesiologist has his own preference when it comes to administering the anesthetic. In some hospitals, the epidural is placed on a pump that you can safely control.

Many couples are concerned about becoming paralyzed from using an epidural. The short answer is that it is highly unlikely. The needle is not inserted into an area that can cause a real problem. Paralysis usually results when the spinal nerve is severed. A needle prick such as the one that happens as a result of an epidural will not sever a nerve. A needle can hit the nerve, but the worst thing that can happen is that you will inadvertently kick the person in front of you. Occasionally, if the epidural needle goes into the dura, it can leave a hole when removed. In that case, spinal fluid can leak out, causing a spinal headache - which is like a migraine - lasting for three to four days. A spinal headache occurs in about 1 in 30 women and can be taken care of with a procedure called a blood patch. A small amount of blood is taken from your arm and placed in the hole created by the spinal needle. The blood will then clot and plug up the hole, eliminating the headache. If left alone, the headache will go away in a few days. A postpartum woman walking around with a spinal headache and a newborn baby is not a fun situation, but it is not paralysis!

Spinal Anesthesia

This is the most common anesthesia when it comes to scheduled or planned C-sections. The reason for this is because spinals give greater pain relief and numbness, which is necessary for surgery. The procedure is the same as the epidural but it is often quicker and the needle passes through the dura. The possibility of a spinal headache is more common with spinal anesthesia.

Paralysis as a result of an epidural is incredibly rare and usually only happens when the woman suffers from a blood clotting disorder – information your doctor should already know about you. In my many years of teaching, no one I have worked with has ever left the hospital in a wheelchair, which is a pretty good statistic! If you still have questions about this issue, please speak with your doctor or midwife. It's better to have your fears addressed and allayed before labor begins.

Walking Epidurals

The difference between an epidural and a walking epidural is the type of medication used. In a regular epidural, an anesthetic is used, which results in the complete numbing of the legs. A walking epidural, however, is a mixture of medications called a cocktail, but bears very little resemblance to a Martini. With this type of epidural, you can still walk, urinate, move around and, best of all, push the baby out. The only issue with the walking epidural is its limited effectiveness, which sometimes necessitates an additional regular epidural. If this happens toward the end of labor, it might not be feasible to hook up the epidural. There is also the possible side effect of itching throughout the body. The best thing to do is to speak to your doctor.

The question I get asked more than any other is, "When is the best time to get an epidural?" I'm thinking, "Here I am trying to teach normal birth and all you guys want to hear about is epidurals!" Well, my answer is always: "Wait until you need it." Of course that may mean a different time for each person because of pain threshold differences. My advice if you're going to use an epidural, is to move your labor forward as much as possible by walking. When you can't walk anymore, it may be time to get the epidural.

From my years as an obstetrical nurse, epidurals seem to have the best outcome when administered at five centimeters or beyond, when we're sure that active labor has really begun.

If you are experiencing out-of-control pain, then ignore what I've just said and go ahead and get the epidural as soon as it is feasible. Sometimes women find that they can use the analgesic to control the pain until they are five centimeters and then switch over to an epidural, which is completely possible.

If you can manage the pain, there is really no reason to rush to get an epidural. Some institutions push epidurals because they think you will have a better childbirth experience. However, the sooner you take it, the higher the chance that your labor could be compromised or disrupted which could lead to a C-section.

I often hear the question, "Is it ever too late to get an epidural?" The answer is, "Yes." Since it takes about 15 minutes to administer an epidural and the same amount of time for it to take affect, there may not be enough time to make the procedure worthwhile for a rapidly progressing labor. If you are lucky enough to have a fast labor, remember to use your comfort measures. You might be surprised at how well you can manage without the medication.

General Anesthesia

The best thing about general anesthesia is that it is fast acting. If there's an emergency situation and the doctor needs to get the baby out quickly, an epidural will take too long to administer. The worst thing about general anesthesia is that it affects the baby immediately. Babies born when the mother is put under general anesthesia are usually slower to breathe than other babies, which is why we get the baby out quickly. In addition, the mother has a slower recovery and cannot participate in the birth in any way. She usually has a tube inserted down her throat for an airway, which means that she'll wake up with a scratched and sore throat. When she wakes up, about an hour later, she might suffer from nausea. Unfortunately, the partner can't participate in this birth, either. However, if time is of the essence, general anesthesia is a godsend.

In the old days, women who needed C-sections were often given the choice between an epidural and general anesthesia. Now, C-sections are usually performed under an epidural/spinal unless it is an emergency.

Pitocin

Pitocin is the synthetic form of Oxytocin, which is the hormone that contracts your uterus. It is used to induce or enhance labor. The word "enhance" sounds gentle, but the drug not only enhances labor, it also enhances pain. Labor contractions are much stronger when labor is manually induced. My labor with my twins was induced, and I can tell you that those contractions were MIGHTY PAINFUL.

The good news is that when you are on Pitocin, you don't have to wait to be five centimeters dilated before getting an epidural. All you need to do is to wait for the first bad contraction and then they will place the epidural. The epidural will work even if you are only one centimeter dilated.

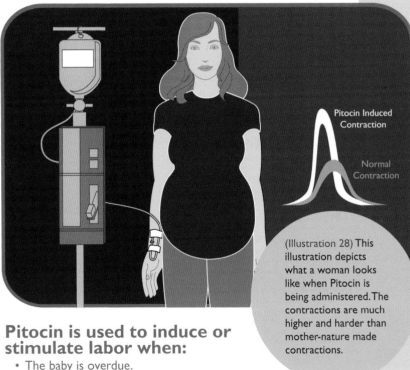

Pitocin Induced Contraction

Normal Contraction

(Illustration 28) This illustration depicts what a woman looks like when Pitocin is being administered. The contractions are much higher and harder than mother-nature made contractions.

Pitocin is used to induce or stimulate labor when:

- The baby is overdue.
- The baby is getting too big for a vaginal delivery.
- You've had an epidural and your labor has slowed down.
- Your labor has stalled for some reason.
- Your water/membranes have broken and you don't experience contractions.

How is Pitocin administered? You will be hooked up to a monitor and then Pitocin is given in measured doses through an IV and a pump. The dose starts at a low level and then gradually increases to almost imitate a real labor. But while Mother Nature takes about 20 hours to complete labor, Pitocin will cut this time in half, mostly 12 hours from start to finish. Pitocin can take up to three hours to begin working, but when it does, the contractions are more painful than natural labor because there is no gradual build-up. Pitocin tends to bypass early labor and create booming contractions right away. This is why we in the profession call this an "F&F labor", short for "fast & furious".

As wonderful a drug as Pitocin is to stimulate a stalled labor or to get the whole process underway, sometimes it doesn't work. If your cervix has already begun to efface and dilate, then the chances are good that Pitocin will successfully induce labor. If the cervix hasn't dilated or effaced, the odds are that the induction will fail. And if an induction fails, the only other choice is a C-section. Pitocin can also cause a "tetanic" contraction, meaning that the contraction never stops. In rare cases if this happens, your uterus could rupture, so the drug has to be turned off immediately which means that labor will most likely stop. Sometimes the doctor will try the induction again at a lower dose, but many times a C-section will be the result.

There is a drug called Cervidil, a gel that can be placed in the cervix prior to a Pitocin induction, which will sometimes soften the cervix and help the Pitocin work more effectively.

In discussions of induction, I would be remiss if I didn't mention "convenience inductions". This is an increasingly troublesome phenomenon in which women with their doctor's urging will be induced to the convenience of the physician or woman herself. As mentioned in the six care practices, and it bears repeating, "Labor should happen on its own."

When you choose to have a baby on a certain day for your convenience, you are messing with Mother Nature. I can tell you from experience, the chances of having a surgical birth following a convenience induction is greatly increased especially with a first baby. If you have a say about this, stick to your guns and wait for labor to happen on its own. Your body knows when it's ready. Trust your body to go into labor and the outcome will be much better.

FORCEPS

www.laughandlearn.com

Forceps look like salad tongs. They have a terrible reputation because of the way they were used over 40 years ago. Back then, when a baby got stuck in the narrowest area of the pelvic region, 0 (zero) station, the doctor would use forceps to pull the baby out, often resulting in damage to the baby. This was called a "high forceps delivery". Nowadays, we only perform "mid-to-low forceps deliveries", which means the baby's head must be visible in the vagina at a +2 or +3 station.

There are two reasons forceps are used. The first is maternal exhaustion. Before I delivered my twins, I couldn't really understand how a woman could get so tired that she couldn't keep pushing. Now, I understand it completely! After ten long hours of labor followed by two hours of pushing, I was completely exhausted and thought I would give up. But with some great cheering from my labor nurses, I was able to keep pushing. The second reason is fetal distress, which is a term we use whenever the heart rate of the baby goes down. If the baby's head is at the opening, it's sometimes too late to perform a C-section, so forceps are used.

In most cases an episiotomy needs to be performed first to make room for the forceps. The doctor will then place the forceps in the hollow below the cheekbones and pull the baby out. Often, but not always, there will be a little bruise around the cheeks and on either side of the forehead. Years ago, babies might actually get dents in their foreheads because they couldn't see where they were placing the forceps. Luckily, that doesn't happen any more!

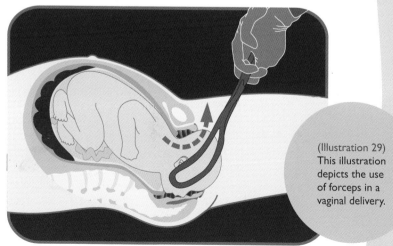

(Illustration 29) This illustration depicts the use of forceps in a vaginal delivery.

The vacuum extractor is an alternative to forceps. It is a suction cup that we place on top of the head to extract the baby. Many of my couples over the years have asked me, "Will this make my baby's head look like a cone head?" The answer is, "No!" Bumps and bulges on the baby's head occur in most vaginal deliveries as a result of the shape of the vagina, even when forceps or the vacuum extractor haven't been used. If a baby is sitting in the vagina for any length of time, the head will elongate to fit the space. Don't worry. The head goes back to a normal shape, usually within a short period of time.

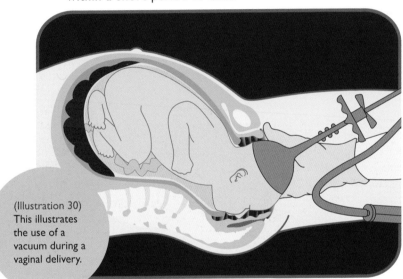

(Illustration 30) This illustrates the use of a vacuum during a vaginal delivery.

Sometimes the vacuum doesn't work. When the baby is still inside the mother, he is surrounded by water, which creates a vacuum from inside the uterus. When the vacuum is placed on the baby's head and the machine is turned on, a tug of war will ensue and the vacuum might pop off the baby's head. Usually the doctor will try it a couple of times and if it doesn't work, forceps are used. Forceps tend to be the more successful instrument, but parents often prefer the vacuum extractor because it's not as invasive as the forceps. It is made out of plastic, and it's placed on the child's head and not on their face. FYI: An episiotomy is also necessary when using the vacuum extractor.

www.laughandlearn.com

External Monitors

External monitors are used to intermittently monitor labor contractions and the fetal heart rate during labor. They can be taken on and off. One disk of the monitor is called a pressure transducer and it is placed on the top of the mother's belly. This disk measures the contraction pattern. Every time you have a contraction, it pushes up against the belly and creates a wave that is measured on the monitor. The other disk is placed further down on the mother's body and it measures the baby's heart rate. The fetal heart monitor measures sound waves so the problem is if the baby moves, the monitor loses information as the heart moves out of range. When this happens, internal monitors are sometimes inserted. In some hospitals as well as with some doctors, continuous monitoring is standard practice, which means you remain on the external monitors continuously throughout your labor. If you use any form of medication in labor you will likely be continuously monitored.

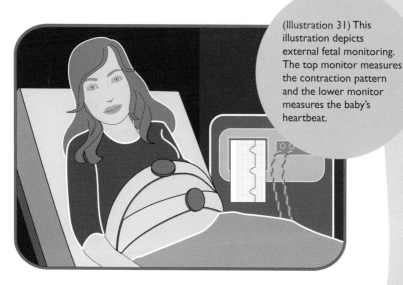

(Illustration 31) This illustration depicts external fetal monitoring. The top monitor measures the contraction pattern and the lower monitor measures the baby's heartbeat.

In some hospitals as well as with some doctors, continuous monitoring is standard practice, which means you remain on the external monitors continuously throughout your labor.

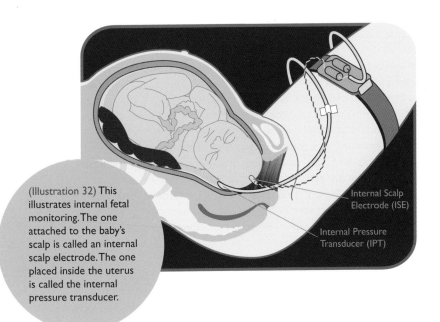

(Illustration 32) This illustrates internal fetal monitoring. The one attached to the baby's scalp is called an internal scalp electrode. The one placed inside the uterus is called the internal pressure transducer.

Internal Scalp Electrode (ISE)

Internal Pressure Transducer (IPT)

In my experience, intermittent monitoring is the better choice. Taking the monitors off in intervals gives you more mobility and in-turn a better chance to labor successfully. Once again, another care practice: freedom of movement. In all the studies that have been done concerning this subject, there are more Cesareans performed when a woman is continuously monitored. It has also been discovered that there has been no significant difference in outcome for the baby when comparing the two. What that means to you, is that your baby will probably do better without all that extra intervention and your chances for a normal birth are increased. This is one of those things you should discuss with your caregiver before your labor, so there will be no surprises when you come in for your delivery.

Internal Monitors

Internal monitors are used to continuously monitor your labor and are used when you are experiencing labor problems or complications. The type of monitor that is connected to the baby is called a scalp electrode. It has a wire on top that looks like a corkscrew. The monitor is inserted into the vagina and gently embedded into the baby's scalp. The wires are attached to a leg band on the mother's thigh. This monitor goes everywhere the baby goes and provides accurate information about the baby to the medical team. Most parents are shocked when they think about having a wire stuck into their baby's scalp, but keep in mind there are no nerve endings in the top layer of skin, so the baby will not feel any pain. Also, the area where the electrode was implanted will scab and peel off shortly after birth. I use an analogy to make this more palatable to my couples: Remember when you were young, and you learned you could put a straight pin through the top layer of skin on your finger without pain? This is the same thing. Keep in mind that this type of monitor is only used when there is a problem with the baby's heart rate. If there is no problem, an internal monitor will not be necessary.

There is another type of internal monitor that is called an internal pressure transducer, which measures the strength of the contractions against the baby's head. To connect this monitor, a tube is inserted directly into the mother's uterus. The strength of the contractions can be an issue, especially when Pitocin is used to enhance or induce labor, making this monitor sometimes necessary.

The types of monitors used depend on the risk level of the pregnancy and the decision of the doctor. If everything's going well with your labor, there's no reason to use internal monitors – the external monitors will work just fine. In my case, I was induced with Pitocin but was not connected to internal monitors.

As you can see, this information can be quite daunting, but that's the point. You will feel much more informed and prepared to make the decisions you will need to make if faced with these choices. In my classes, I often find this is the toughest content to teach because it can be scary. However, you can take a slow deep breath now – we're almost finished.

If you want to give birth as naturally as possible it is important to speak with your caregiver and make sure your wishes be known.

Chapter 6

One of my goals as a childbirth educator is to inform and
educate women on how to avoid an unnecessary C-Section.

— Sheri Bayles

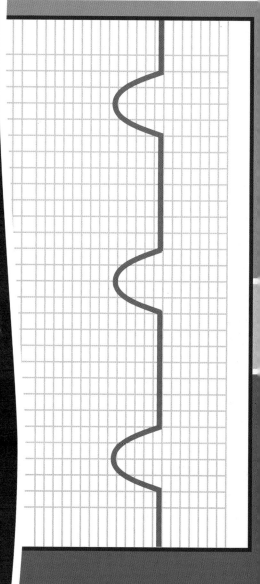

Cesarean
Delivery,
Post-Op C/S,
and
Postpartum
Vaginal
Delivery

In the last chapter I discussed the exceptions to a normal birth. We in the field have noticed that the more the medical staff intervenes during labor, the more likely you will experience the "cascade of interventions" which often leads to a Cesarean delivery. Because of this, I can't stress enough how important staying on your feet and working with gravity is to producing the best possible outcome.

Let me explain. Once you choose to take medications for labor, you will need an IV for hydration, followed by a blood pressure cuff to monitor your blood pressure, then an urinary catheter will be placed into your bladder, along with continuous monitoring. Most likely your labor will slow down from the combination of meds and sitting on a bed, so Pitocin will probably be added to the IV.

In my experience, this is when the Pitocin is least effective, and because you do not progress, down the hall you go for a Cesarean delivery.

CESAREAN DELIVERY

Ten Indicators for a C-section

1. The baby's too big: Which is called CPD, meaning "Cephalopelvic Disproportion". When discussing this reason with some midwives, they often tell me that this can be avoided by keeping the mother as upright as possible along with squatting and sitting on a birthing ball. If a mom's pelvis is wide enough, the baby will descend. There are of course those really big babies, that won't fit through, but they tend to be the minority.

2. Fetal Distress: When the baby's heart rate goes down for any reason, all hell breaks loose in the birthing room. When the baby is in fetal distress, an alarm goes off and many people come running. The nurses will immediately turn you from your left side (which is the best position to provide the baby with enough oxygen) onto your right side to reposition the baby. If the cord has slipped between the baby and a bone, the repositioning will

do the trick. Next, an oxygen mask will be placed on you to raise the level of oxygen to the baby. If these two measures don't work, a "scalp pH" will be performed by going into the vagina, pricking the baby's scalp and drawing blood. The blood will be analyzed to determine the baby's oxygen level. If the level is low, that is often grounds for having an emergency C-section. In my experience this most often happens when you have an epidural. Since you are not moving around, the baby tends to stay in one place and the baby's cord may become compromised.

www.laughandlearn.com

3. The Baby is in the Wrong Position: Such as breech (bottom down) or transverse (baby is sideways across the belly). The correct position is called vertex, which means head down. In years past, a breech vaginal delivery was very common. However due to the fear of a difficult delivery, most caregivers today resort to a Cesarean delivery.

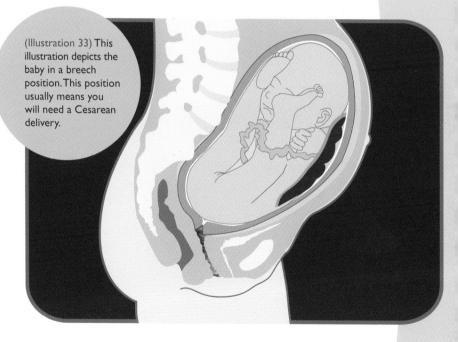

(Illustration 33) This illustration depicts the baby in a breech position. This position usually means you will need a Cesarean delivery.

4. Placenta Previa: When the placenta is located low in the uterus and is blocking the opening of the cervix. This is often determined early in the pregnancy with the use of a sonogram.

5. Placenta Abruptia: When the placenta separates from the uterine wall while the baby is still in the uterus. It's a rare condition that causes extreme pain and heavy bleeding. This is one of the few occasions when you should go immediately to the closest emergency room, and I mean closest hospital, even if your regular hospital is only 30 minutes away. Not only are you in danger due to hemorrhaging, but the baby is also losing oxygen. Some possible indicators of placenta abruptia are women over forty having a first baby, hypertension in pregnancy and problems with the placenta during pregnancy. This one sounds pretty scary, but as I stated earlier, it is a rare occurrence for a healthy woman.

6. **Prolapsed Cord:** When the cord slips down in front of the baby's head. Remember to sit down when you break your water. This will help prevent the cord from slipping down. This is more common with second pregnancies than first because the baby tends to engage later in the labor on a second go round.

7. **Failure to progress:** When contractions are occurring but the cervix is not opening even after Pitocin is administered. This is most common after an epidural is administered too early in the labor.

8. **Failed induction:** When labor is induced but doesn't work, a C-section is often the only option.

9. **Hypertension during pregnancy:** High blood pressure can create many complications during labor, so a C-section is the best route.

10. **Herpes:** As long as you don't have a lesion that is shedding at the time of delivery, a C-section isn't necessary. Most often your doctor or midwife knows the situation with this condition before labor starts.

What Happens During a C-section

Unlike a vaginal delivery where shaving isn't necessary, you will be shaved from the top of your tummy straight down to the top of your legs for a C-section. A catheter will be placed in your bladder to keep it empty during surgery. The medical staff will place a blood pressure cuff on one of your arms and an IV in the other. Your arms will be put on boards so that they cannot move and affect the sterile field, which is the area below your chest. A drape is placed across your chest to mark the sterile field but also to block you and your partners' vision. In most cases, you'll be anesthetized by an epidural or spinal, with a much stronger dosage than that used for vaginal deliveries.

Normally, your obstetrician will perform the surgery, which takes about an hour – five minutes to cut, and 45 minutes to stitch you up. She'll make a horizontal (left to right) incision across the pubic hairline that is called a "bikini cut". This is the more common procedure because only with a horizontal incision can you have a VBAC (Vaginal Birth After Cesarean) with your next baby. With an up and down incision the abdominal muscle won't be able to tolerate a future labor. In the old days, surgeons made only vertical (up and down) incisions, called "Classical C's", which are sometimes necessary nowadays depending on the placement of the placenta. We used to have a saying, "Once a C-section always a C-section". With horizontal incisions, this no longer applies.

Partners are often allowed to be in the operating room as long as you sit down next to your wife's head. The medical staff wants to eliminate the possibility that you might faint if you watch the surgery. However, in some institutions, partners are allowed to stand and even take pictures if the medical staff agrees.

After the baby is lifted out of you, the pediatrician (who has been called in from the medical staff) will APGAR the baby. Then the nurses will perform all the procedures we discussed in Chapter 3, like wiping the baby down, putting Erythromycin Ointment in the baby's eyes, placing an identification bracelet on the baby, and giving the baby an injection of Vitamin K to help with clotting. The next step involves taking the placenta out and then the obstetrician begins stitching you up layer by layer. Sometimes the doctor will give you some form of sedative so that you can remain calm and relaxed during the rest of the surgery.

After the delivery, you will then be taken to the recovery room. Depending on hospital policy, the baby might go with you or be taken to the nursery. In an ideal world, the baby would be with you in the recovery room so that you can breastfeed as soon as possible after birth. Again, one of the six care practices: mother and baby should not be separated after birth. Since some hospitals don't allow this, you should find out ahead of time the hospital's policy.

While in recovery, you will be hooked up to an IV, still have the blood pressure cuff on and the catheter will still be in your bladder. You will probably feel shaky and shivery, which is very common after any surgery. The nurses will place extra blankets on you and you'll stay in recovery for about two hours. Partners are usually allowed to follow the new mothers through this whole process. After two hours, you'll be moved to your postpartum room and your baby will join you.

Pain Medication After a C-Section

Unlike a vaginal delivery where you are up and about almost immediately, after a C-section you will have to stay in bed for 18-24 hours. You will also experience pain from the surgery for which you will be given medication. A few different drugs could be:

Doramorph: A morphine derivative that is delivered into your epidural space and lasts about one to eight hours. It's very effective at taking the pain away, but you may experience some nausea and vomiting. From my experience, its' biggest side effect is that it causes itching. Benadryl is used to counteract this.

PCA (patient-controlled analgesia): You are in control of the pain medication, usually morphine. With a push of a button, you self-administer (yippee!) your own pain medication through an intravenous pump. Again, the pump is self-regulating, so no worries about over-medicating. This type of medication doesn't disrupt your breastfeeding because the amount of morphine that passes through the breast is minimal. PCA is wonderful because you moms won't have to wait for someone to come and give you more pain medication. It puts you in control of your recovery, which is very empowering after a C-section. The one drawback to morphine is that it may make you feel very groggy and "loopy". In this state, you may have difficulty getting the breastfeeding started since you feel like you are in the ozone. You will receive pain medication as long as you need it. Most women come off the PCA after two days and then use oral medication to control the pain.

Oral medications: Many hospitals only use oral medications such as Percocet for pain relief after a C-section. This medication often gives just the right amount of pain relief without a groggy feeling. It is also perfectly safe to breastfeed with this medication. As far as I'm concerned this is the best choice for mothers following a surgical birth.

C-Section Recovery

After the initial 18-24 hours of bed rest, the urinary catheter will come out, but the IV will stay in until you are ready for solid food. Most insurance companies cover a four-night stay in the hospital after a C-section and two nights for a vaginal delivery. Most often this is how long you will stay. Please keep in mind that after a C-section it takes two weeks to feel good, four weeks to feel marvelous, and six weeks to feel like you've never had surgery.

Here Are Some Tips to Make Your Recovery Easier For You:
1. If possible, get a private room
In most hospitals, if you have a private room your partner can stay over with you and the baby. Having your partner with you after giving birth is not only very comforting, it is very practical. After a C-section, every movement hurts and you will need help getting to the bathroom, picking up the baby and moving the baby from breast to breast. Keep in mind that a C-section is abdominal surgery and your muscles have been cut or separated. It's a bit similar to the feeling you have the day after doing 50 sit-ups when you haven't exercised in years. The more help you have in the days and weeks after a C-section, the better you will feel.

2. Sip warm water or chamomile tea after moving to your postpartum room
During a C-section you are cut open and air gets into the bowels and shuts them down. After a C-section, the nursing staff will ask you repeatedly whether you have passed gas. When I worked as a nurse on the floors, I must have asked this question at least 3000 times. Every once in a while, the patient wasn't sure what I was asking, so I had to use the more common terms and ask, "Have you farted?" At that point, my question was clearly understood and

I would get a bright "Yes!" in reply. I was trying to be delicate but instead I was just misunderstood. The reason this is done is to determine whether your bowels are operating again so you can be given solid food. If the bowels aren't functioning, the stomach will throw up whatever solid food you eat. Throwing up after abdominal surgery is not a good idea. Until the bowels are working, you will be given small amounts of clear liquid.

For years patients would always get "sips and chips" after a C-section, meaning little sips of water and ice chips. Over the course of my nursing career, however, I discovered that most women were so parched they literally inhaled the ice chips as fast as they could, which sends a lot of cold fluid right into the already cramped bowel which makes their condition even worse. I discovered that if the patient instead sipped small quantities of warm water, chamomile or peppermint tea, the bowel opened up faster and the mom's recovery went more quickly.

When the ice chips arrive, thank the nurse very much, wait until she leaves and then have your partner dump them in the sink and head out to get a cup of warm water. Most hospitals have microwave ovens so this shouldn't be a problem. If you want chamomile tea, fine, but don't gulp it. Sip it - put it down for a little while - sip it - and put it back down again. I guarantee that if you do this for the first two days and never touch an ice chip, you will pass gas within 48 hours with no gas pains. I have had many women over the years thank me for this advice because it works so well.

3. Don't invite your relatives to visit for the first 24 hours
After a C-section, you won't feel like having visitors for at least 24 hours so give yourself a well-deserved rest and ask your relatives to wait just a little while longer before coming to the hospital! I know, I know. Some of you are saying, "But you don't know my mother-in-law!" Believe me, I actually do. If the relatives insist, make the visits short and sweet. After the first 24-48 hours, you will be feeling much better and will be more able to deal with them.

To pass gas faster following a cesarean delivery, sip only warm, clear liquids, like tea or broth.

4. Get out of bed and stay out of bed

Most women do not want to move after abdominal surgery. However the longer you stay in bed, the longer it takes for your muscles to work. You will find it is easier to move around if you sit in a chair with arms, since that will give you leverage when you are getting up and down. Climbing in and out of bed is difficult at best, so staying out of bed during the day will help with healing and getting your bowels to function faster.

5. Make sure to have help when you go home for at least a week or two

This piece of advice is very important because after a C-section you won't be able to handle everything by yourself when you get home. For the first two weeks following surgery, to help with the healing of your incision,

You should:

- **NOT** lift anything heavier than your baby.

- **NOT** move furniture, which includes moving a rocking chair or pushing a bassinet on wheels across the room.

- **NOT** climb stairs more than once a day. And when you do climb stairs, it's one step at a time.

- **NOT** drive a car! Because you use your abdominal muscles when you step on the gas or brake pedals.

So that's why you need the help. Even if you're completely sure you're going to have a vaginal delivery, please have a back-up plan so you're covered. Think about who you would like to have with you when you get home from the hospital. If you have to hire someone, do it. Don't ask your mother or mother-in-law unless you have a really good relationship with her and she's a real helper.

To review, when recovering from a cesarean, it usually takes a full six weeks to recover. As far as I'm concerned, it's not the delivery that is a problem, it's the recovery. I am often asked if there is any way to absolutely avoid a cesarean. My best advice has always been, wait at home as long as possible, because the sooner you enter a hospital setting, the faster multiple interventions will occur. Trust that inner wisdom to help you make the right decisions!!

Your Uterus

After you have the baby, your uterus does not contract back to its original shape for about six weeks, which means you might look as if you're six months pregnant for a little while. Try not to be insulted if someone unfamiliar with this childbirth fact asks you if you're pregnant shortly after you've had your baby, or what I call "foot-in-mouth visitors disease". It's usually some man from the office, a single guy who has never seen a postpartum woman in his life. He comes up to your partner after seeing your belly and whispers, "I thought she had the baby!" My response would be, "Just leave the gift on the bed, and get the heck out of here!" Keep a few maternity clothes handy and do not despair. Your waistline will re-appear after about three months (maybe longer if you're over 35).

Your Breasts

For the first two to three days after you have given birth, your breasts will be soft and produce colostrum (a precursor to the milk), which is a yellowish clear fluid. It is the perfect nutrition for your baby and protects them against infection. On the third or fourth day (sometimes longer if you have had a C-section) the milk comes in and the breasts sometimes become hard and red, which we call engorgement. For some of you, your breasts may feel like you're carting around watermelons. For others, you may breeze through this. Engorgement usually takes 48 hours to go away and can be uncomfortable. The best way to alleviate engorgement is to breastfeed often, apply moist warm packs to the breasts or take a warm shower before feedings. Use ice packs on the breasts immediately after the feedings. If you're not planning on breastfeeding, wear a tight bra and use ice packs for 48 hours and the engorgement will go away by itself.

Perineal Discomfort or Pain Due to Episiotomy or Tearing

After childbirth, you might experience pain or discomfort in your perineum (the area around the vagina and rectum) resulting from an episiotomy or tearing. The stitches are dissolvable and the wound takes about two weeks to heal. The nursing staff at the hospital or birthing center will advise you about how to handle this discomfort. Most hospitals give patients a bottle filled with warm water to squirt over the perineal area after going to the bathroom to keep the area clean. Ice packs are often used immediately following your delivery to reduce any swelling from the pushing. I also recommend sitting on a sitz bath. Ahh … what is that? It's a small plastic bowl filled with warm water that is placed onto the toilet bowl. Sitting your hips and buttocks in the warm water can be very soothing. At this point you are not allowed to take a tub bath, so this helps with perineal discomfort.

Hemorrhoids

As if perineal pain isn't bad enough, you might also have pain and discomfort thanks to hemorrhoids. Hemorrhoids are enlarged veins outside the anus, which look like small mushrooms and are the result of pressure on the rectum caused by bearing down to push the baby out. In my case, I never had a hemorrhoid in my life until I had my sons. Ever! After the epidural wore off, I remember feeling pain and saying to my doctor, "What the heck did you do to me down there?" She replied that she had done an episiotomy and that I had hemorrhoids that would heal in a few weeks. Sounds simple enough. But let me tell you that having a bowel movement when you have hemorrhoids is almost worse than giving birth. When I got home and attempted my first bowel movement, I remember shouting to my husband on the other side of the bathroom door, "I want an epidural for this!" But not every woman gets hemorrhoids from a vaginal delivery.

Sitting after Childbirth

I taught classes in the hospital to mothers that had given birth and watching them try to sit down was quite amusing. Since I have given birth, I can now relate to these new moms on a very personal level and have earned the right to chuckle.

Picture this: A parade of postpartum women who look like Charlie Chaplin as they walk down the hall to class. Their feet are as far apart as they can be and still walk. As they enter the classroom, they lean up against the door wondering how they are going to sit down through a full hour class on how to give their newborn a bath.

The mothers who have given birth vaginally have no idea how they are going to sit. They stare at the chairs as if they are foreign objects. They walk around them trying desperately to get the inspiration or the courage they will need to finally sit. Suddenly, they have an epiphany. They place their hands on the armrest, cross one leg over the other, and somehow manage to sit on their hip. Yes, they are now leaning into the woman sitting next to them, but this is not a time to debate "personal space" issues.

On the other hand, the mothers who have had C-sections do what I call the "parallel park". They back themselves into the chairs and sit down with their legs as far apart as possible. Breaking every rule of ladylike behavior, these women sigh as their bottoms hit the chair, wondering how they are going to make it through the next six weeks.

Having been there, I know that each and every one of these bottom-challenged women is actually a superhero-in-disguise who will someday look back on all of this and laugh.

Lochia

Lochia is the discharge that comes out of your vagina after giving birth. It is a mixture of the uterine lining and blood. Over several weeks, the lochia progressively changes color and consistency and then it stops altogether.

- For about a week, the discharge is moderate and red in color.
- The next week, the lochia is brown and spotting.
- The third week, the lochia is pink in color.
- And finally, about a month after delivering your baby, the discharge is white and creamy. This is the time that your doctor or midwife will usually want to see you back in the office.

Within two to six weeks after birth, the doctor or midwife wants to check you out internally to make sure that your cervix is closing up and the bleeding is subsiding. The progression of the bleeding is a great gauge to determine how well you're healing. If your discharge has progressed to brown and then goes back to red, you're overexerting yourself and should slow down! Up until that visit with your doctor, you will follow the hospital discharge instructions that are quite simple: "NOTHING GOES UP THE VAGINA FOR FOUR TO SIX WEEKS!" No intercourse, douching, tampons, tub baths or swimming!

I once had a woman a day after giving birth ask me to tell her husband that she couldn't have sex for four to six months, instead of four to six weeks. Until I had my twins, I couldn't understand why she would have wanted me to do that. The minute my epidural wore off and I felt those hemorrhoids, I understood completely. Partners, be patient. The more understanding you are to your spouse, the sooner she'll feel like her old self.

www.laughandlearn.com

Weight Loss

The bad news: It's hard to sit down. The good news: On the day you deliver, you'll lose 9-13 pounds! In the next week, you could lose up to about five pounds of water weight, which means that if you experienced swelling during your pregnancy, your hands and ankles will be normal again! If you are nursing, you could lose another 10 pounds rather quickly, which is another upside to nursing. During my pregnancy with twins, I gained 35 pounds, which thankfully was on the low side. Within two weeks, I took off 32 pounds. My doctor was shocked. I reminded her that I was breastfeeding twins, which meant that I was burning 1,000 to 2,000 calories a day! And for you foodaholics, I was consuming 4000 calories a day to make up for it. For me, breastfeeding was better than going to the gym every day for two hours. Some women lose weight initially when they start breastfeeding, but then the weight loss levels off. If you've gained over 25 pounds during a pregnancy, you'll have to exert more effort to lose the weight down the road. But to be honest, breastfeeding my babies was the best weight loss program I have ever been on!

Postpartum Blues

During pregnancy, a woman's hormone levels increase dramatically to nurture new life. After the baby is born, these levels drop suddenly and postpartum blues can result. The most common symptom of the blues is weepiness. You'll look at your new baby and begin to cry or you might just begin crying for no reason at all. This is completely normal. Be kind to yourself! If you feel that your blues are more like depression, talk to your doctor about it immediately. Therapy and antidepressants can work wonders and many antidepressant drugs will not affect your ability to breastfeed.

Partners, please understand that this is normal and should go away within a few weeks. The best way to respond to a weepy new mother

CHAPTER SIX: CESAREAN DELIVERY, POST-OP C/S, & POSTPARTUM VAGINAL DELIVERY **123** is simply to show compassion and understanding. Trying to talk a postpartum woman out of crying is a waste of time! Go with the flow and do your very best to help out as much as possible with the baby. A few boxes of tissues casually placed around the house may also help!

Sleep Deprivation

Within two to four weeks after a vaginal delivery, you will feel great! But by then, the effects of sleep deprivation might start setting in. Most newborn babies eat every few hours, right through the night. While they also sleep a lot, sometimes it's not at night! The hardest aspect of parenting is that it is a 24-hour a day job, even when you're working outside the home. Sleeping while the baby sleeps is a good plan right after the baby is born and some parents swear by sleep-sharing or co-sleeping (sleeping with the baby either in your bed or in a bedside bassinet) as a great way to help keep sleep deprivation to a minimum. I also recommend adding a bottle to the baby's diet after the breastfeeding has become well established. This way your partner can take a feeding in the late evening hours and you can get a full five hours of sleep. I discuss this fully in my *Laugh and Learn About Breastfeeding* DVD. Investigating your options and discussing your feelings before the baby is born can help you feel a bit more prepared for your new lifestyle with baby.

It usually takes two weeks to feel good following a vaginal delivery.

Conclusion

There is no greater joy than the day
your baby enters the world.

— Sheri Bayles

Some final words on the
current state of childbirth today,

how it affects you and

what you can do about it.

In general, the state of childbirth is much better then it has been in the past. We know a lot more then we did even a short time ago. In the 23 years I have been teaching, I have seen good and bad, but have seen much change for the better. The most important issue today is that birth is too often treated as a medical procedure instead of a natural and normal process. In this book we have reviewed the things you can do and the things you should avoid during your labor to help you decrease medical intervention, which often leads to a surgical birth. As a childbirth educator, I am concerned that the number of C-sections in America is climbing at an alarming rate. When I started teaching in 1986, the C-section rate was hovering around 22 percent nationwide. It is now running 30-35 percent, depending on the hospital. It has dramatically increased to the detriment of all involved. Eighty-seven percent of all healthy young pregnant women should be able to deliver their babies vaginally, so why are we seeing such a high rate? In fact, The World Health Organization has set a future goal to decrease the number of C-sections to 10-15 percent worldwide. One of my goals as a childbirth educator is to inform and educate women on what they can do to avoid an unnecessary C-section. I would also like to see the birthing experience given back to the mother. After all, it is her experience and one she will remember for the rest of her life.

The best way I know to accomplish this goal is to make sure you know your options and know what you are up against. If you are trying to achieve a vaginal delivery along with the possibility of a natural delivery (which means no medications involved), I want you to know what to do. I also want you to understand the childbirth process so you can make the best choices for yourself.

Throughout this book I have talked to you about having a normal childbirth, which is both how Mother Nature intended it and often provides the best outcome for both mother and baby.

Today a normal birth is defined as a vaginal delivery with as little intervention as possible. Routine hospital interventions can range from IV's, monitors, medications, forceps, vacuum, catheters and anything that ends up on or in a woman's body during labor. The more interventions involved, the less the woman's body works naturally, which can ultimately lead to a surgical birth.

In this book, I have taught you about the pros and cons of those interventions, so when you are faced with these issues, you can make an informed decision without fear.

So how can you take this knowledge and make it work for you? Well, the most important thing for you to do is to start a dialogue with your doctor/midwife about having a normal delivery with as little intervention as possible. The following ideas are helpful when talking with your medical professional:

Make a birth plan: Look at your doctor/midwife as your partner and talk to them about your birth plan. A birth plan is something that lists your wants and wishes. It doesn't always mean it will be followed through, but it's worth writing it up anyway. Come up with five or six really important things that you would like to see happen in labor. While you can't plan a birth, you can ask for things that will help your labor progress normally. Having this discussion with your medical professional before your birth will give you a better idea of what they can accommodate. Bringing your birth plan with you to the hospital is also a good idea.

Education: Read as much about childbirth as you can and educate yourself as much as possible. It has been stated that people spend more time researching a car purchase than educating themselves on having a baby. Here is your opportunity to be well informed. Knowledge is power. The more you know beforehand, the better your decision-making process will be in the future. Knowledge will help you eliminate fear-based decisions.

Throughout this book you have read that labor is a normal process. We in the world of childbirth call it "pain with a purpose." Finding ways to handle pain with labor support and very little medical intervention often leads to a good outcome for both mom and baby. If that happens to you, then I feel that I have accomplished what I have set out to do. If your delivery does not turn out how you would have liked, then the most important thing is that both you and your baby are healthy.

After reading this book you should feel confident, comfortable and above all else, know you can do this!

Personal Author's Note

After spending six weeks with couples in my live class, they are often hesitant about leaving because it means the next time I see them, they will probably have become parents. They also feel that their lives are about to change dramatically, but are not sure just how. For me, as their instructor, it is also bittersweet because I know I have helped them along their journey, but I also know it is time for them to fly on their own. This is how I feel about finishing this book.

Becoming a parent is a wonderful, joyous, challenging and frightening experience. It is also the most difficult job you will ever have, but also the most rewarding. Yes, it's a draining job and you don't always know if you are doing the right thing. But in my opinion, it's the best thing that can happen to you.

My true life began when I became a mother. Bringing my boys into the world brought a whole new meaning to my life. I struggled with sleep deprivation like all new parents do. I often second-guessed my decisions, again, as all new parents do. But I'm also a great deal wiser. Becoming a parent helps you become a grown-up. For some, that may be the most daunting prospect, but my advice is to go with the flow. My second piece of advice is to try and get some sleep. But most importantly, don't worry. Parenting comes with many challenges, but nothing you can't handle.

I've taught you all about your labor and delivery. Now it's time to learn all you can about your baby. Enjoy them as much as possible. Surround yourself with lots of other new parents and you won't feel like you are the only one going through it. My best advice is to keep a sense of humor. Your baby will give you immeasurable joy and laughter. I know, because mine have.

I wish you the very best as you enter the brave new world of parenthood.

—Sheri Bayles

Index

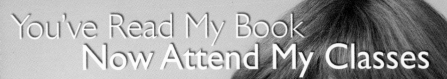
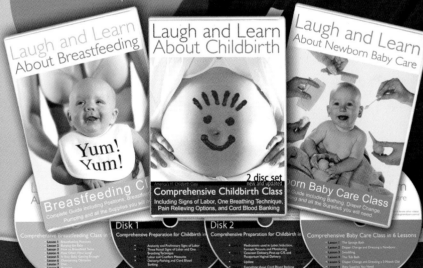